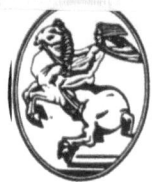

ACTA NEUROCHIRURGICA
SUPPLEMENTUM 26

Gerhard Orf

Critical Resection Length and Gap Distance in Peripheral Nerves

**Experimental
and Morphological Studies**

SPRINGER-VERLAG
WIEN   NEW YORK

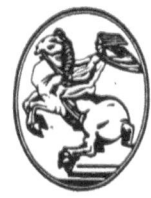

GERHARD ORF, M.D.
Neurosurgical Clinic (Head: Prof. Dr. P. RÖTTGEN) and Institute for
Neuropathology (Head: Prof. Dr. G. KERSTING), Bonn University,
Bonn, Federal Republic of Germany

With 45 Figures

Library of Congress Cataloging in Publication Data. Orf, Gerhard, 1935-   . Critical resection length
and gap distance in peripheral nerves. (Acta neurochirurgica: Supplementum, 26.) Bibliography: p.
1. Nerves, Peripheral-Surgery. 2. Surgery, Experimental. I. Title. II. Series. RD595.073. 617'.483. 78-9048.

ISBN-13:978-3-211-81482-6   e-ISBN-13:978-3-7091-8517-9
DOI: 10.1007/978-3-7091-8517-9

Foreword

The Second World War gave rise to a previously inconceivable number of peripheral nerve injuries. Only later on did these injuries occasion renewed intensive research in this field of neurosurgery. Among the factors which have promoted this development is the operating microscope with more refined surgical techniques. Of course, surgery of peripheral nerve injuries in peacetime is not to be compared with that in wartime. Only rapid wound healing enables a secondary suture to be performed at a favorable time, after about four weeks. Besides in most cases the defect of substance is not as great as in war injuries, in which the so-called "critical resection length" (Seddon) was the cause of the greatest difficulties and constituted the crucial obstacle to good success. The experienced surgeons of the Second World War always knew that the specified dimensions were far too great for the critical resection length. They could only resort to attempting a suture even when there was a great gap between the ends of the nerves. Precise information was not available on direct damage to the axis cylinder or alteration due to vascular factors when stretching the various nerves, above all during the later mobilization of joint decompressions.

In my opinion, the experimental investigations of the author can make a contribution here. The precisely executed and afterwards carefully analyzed experiments appear very likely to be applicable to human conditions as regards their percentages of total nerve length. However, sufficiently verified standard figures are required, above all for the length relations between limbs and nerves. The animal investigations presented show that lesions occur even when stretching a nerve by 2% in the region of narrow passages, whereas without those a 3% stretching is tolerated. However, from 4% stretching onwards there is such extensive nerve damage (primary and secondary) that it no longer appears permissible to bridge these distances with an end-to-end union. A 3% defect in the total nerve length must therefore be generally regarded as the critical resection length for an end-to-end suture. With larger defects, preference should be given to free nerve transplantation.

The studies presented will certainly attract great attention on the part of neurosurgeons and surgeons concerned with peripheral nerve injuries. They will stimulate further studies and applications to human conditions.

P. RÖTTGEN

Contents

VIII   Contents

A. Introduction

The treatment of nerve injuries is one of the still-unsolved problems of neurosurgery, especially, as lesions of this kind generally cause discontinuities and gaps in the nerves. The object of any surgical repair in this field is to produce optimal functional results.

Nearly every end-to-end anastomosis of nerve stumps performed in order to effect the surgical repair of a defect and the anatomical reconstruction of an injured nerve involves stretching of the nerve in question. Consequently, the extent of stretching is proportional to the nerve gap size. If the range of extensibility of a nerve is exceeded beyond a certain degree of strain, its function will be impaired, and its parenchyma will be injured. It is doubtful whether direct neurorrhaphy will be effective under these circumstances, which is why surgeons keep calling for tensionless nerve sutures. Several factors determine the success of a direct end-to-end anastomosis of an injured nerve, the major factor obviously being the size of the gap to be repaired. There are, however, primary and secondary, absolute as well as relative gap sizes.

A primary gap size is defined as existing immediately after an injury has caused a discontinuity. This is the case, for instance, in fresh cuts, resections of neurogenic tumors, neuromas in continuity, neural segments affected by endoneurial fibrosis, etc. It is composed of the combined effects of loss of substance (genuine neural defect) and the retraction of the two nerve ends. Clean cuts, unlike extensive crush injuries, do not produce any further injuries to the parenchyma, so that the distance to which the nerve ends retract from the point of cutting depends exclusively on their natural elasticity. Stoffel (1915), Koschitz-Kosic (1960), Chao, Tsang, and Ts'ui (1962), McQuillan (1965), Petrov and Solarov (1965, 1966), Thomas and Jones (1967), and Millesi (1973) have all reported their findings concerning the gap in the tissue caused by the elastic retraction of nerve ends which commences immediately after a cut. The actual extent of retraction varies. It depends on several factors which include: Length and cross-section of the nerve concerned, the kind of nerve affected, the quantitative composition of its tissue elements and its fascicular structure, the anatomy of its course, the state of the sliding tissue surrounding the nerve, and the type of injury sustained. Additional variations are caused by the position of the joints in the extremity (Stoffel 1915). The separation of the cut ends of a severed nerve reaches its minimum and its maximum according to the position of extreme flexion or extension of the joints, therefore the size of the gap is relative.

A secondary nerve gap is a primary nerve gap enlarged because of freshening of the stumps during secondary operative debridement. To ensure optimal functional repair, a proximal stump whose cross-section appears completely healthy is required for the nerve suture.

It is doubtless difficult to decide on the limit of resection on a purely macro-scopic basis. For this reason, Mackenzie and Woods (1961) even went so far as to use intraoperative histological tests. With the operating microscopes which have come into general use today, it is now possible to determine the transition between pathological and intact nerve cross-sections, with sufficient exactness.

The term "absolute nerve gap" signifies the diastasis between nerve ends which have been adequately freshened back to the healthy tissue. This gap is measured with all joints of the extremity con-cerned in their physiological mid-position. If the absolute nerve gap should be too large to allow tension-free apposition and suture of the nerve ends the diastasis can be reduced by means of several "mani-pulative" measures (Sanders 1942) involving wide operative exposure, mobilization, and transposition of the nerve as well as a favourable position of the extremity for relaxation of the nerve. This means as a rule flexion of the adjacent joints or as a final resort, shortening by osteotomy.

Swan (1941) abandoned the procedure of shortening long bones, which had been recommended by Löbker (1884) and perfected by Kirschner (1917) for the purpose of reducing a nerve diastasis and facilitating end-to-end suture.

In some cases, the application of mobilization is limited, for instance in the immediate neighbourhood of an entry into a hiatus or of a functionally important branch. Severing nutrient vessels in the immediate vicinity may jeopardize the vascular supply to such an extent (Smith 1966) that one puts mobilized nerve sectors nearly on the same level as a free nerve graft (Maurer 1971).

Transposition can be performed only on certain nerves and only in certain anatomical regions. Moreover, it demands a more extensive mobilization of the nerve in question.

The danger of permanent joint contracture is always present while the neighbouring joints are still under postoperative fixation in a position of maximum flexion until the sutured nerve ends are firmly healed. The re-mobilization of joints which is required after immobilization may strain the nerve to the point of rupturing the suture (Spurling 1945, Whitcomb 1946, Woodhall 1959). Both a turnbuckle cast (Highet and Holmes 1943) and the apparatus recommended by Nigst (1955) can be used in an effort to avoid stretch injuries to the nerve by careful, step-by-step mobilization of the affected extremity (Babcock 1927, Cutler and Gross 1936, Seddon 1949, 1954, Scarff 1945, 1958, Naffziger 1921, Björkesten 1947). Forrester-Brown (1921), Platt (1921), Platt and Bristow (1923), Babcock

(1927), Highet and Holmes (1943), and others have reported on obtaining favourable results by these methods which are still widely used today (Nigst 1955, Björkesten 1972, Krenkel 1972, Penzholz 1972, et al.).

The auxiliary measures described above contribute towards either closing or reducing an absolute gap. They do not necessarily have to be applied simultaneously. The following sequence is generally

Table 1. *Critical Resection Lengths of Individual Nerves (cm) Which Can be Offset by Mobilization, Transposition and Flexing of Joints (h = high, m = medium, t = low)*

		SEDDON 1963	NIGST 1962	GRANTHAM &POLLARD 1955	ZACHARY 1954	HIGHET &HOLMES 1943	BABCOCK 1927	FORRESTER -BROWN 1920
Plexus brachialis	h						11,5	
	m							
	t							
Medianus	h	7			7		15	11,5
	m	9		9	8,5	9		
	t	7,5			7		23	16,5
Ulnaris	h	10			10		16	12,5
	m	13	13	9	13	11		
	t	10			10		12,5	16,5
Radialis	h	8			8		15	
	m	8		7	8	6		9—10
	t	7,5			7,5		10,5	
Peronaeus	h	9			9			
	m	9		6	8,8	15	13—15	
	t	9			9			
Tibialis	h	10			11,5			
	m	11	7	9	11	6	13—15	15
	t	7			8			
Ischiadicus	h							
	m			11		8,5	14	10
	t							

adhered to: Mobilization of nerve ends, flexion of joints, transposition. If this should not suffice to close the gap the only remaining method is to force apposition by traction. The strain caused by this measure does not merely affect the locus minoris resistentiae, *i.e.*, the suture itself, but the nerve as well, causing damage due to stretching. Various authors (Forrester-Brown 1920, Babcock 1927, Sanders 1942, Highet and Holmes 1943, Grantham and Pollard 1951, Brooks 1955, Nigst 1962, Seddon 1963; Table 1) have expressed various views on the maximum possible defect which can be dealt with by the auxiliary measures described above so as to allow a direct union of the two nerve ends, *i.e.*, the critical limit or length of resection. Transgressing this limit will jeopardize clinical success.

According to our experience, the critical resection lengths given by the authors above are excessive. The problem is not the length (cm) of the distance bridged by the joining of the two nerve ends but the stress on the joined nerve caused by this process. There is a primary stress caused by applying the suture as well as a post-operative stress caused by the extremity regaining its full mobility after immobilization.

Even if a suture is primarily tension-free the incipient re-innervation is bound to be interfered with later when fixation ends and mobilization of the extremity begins (Millesi 1972).

Early authors, like Baron and Schreiber (1918), Stookey (1922), and Leriche (1940) stated that the postoperative extension of extremities may cause nerve lesions. These statements were corroborated by the experiments of Highet and Sanders (1943).

Optimal clinical results are not ensured merely by re-establishing anatomical continuity nor by a good tensile strength of the circular suture alone. To avoid injuries to the parenchyma caused by stretching or stressing a nerve during reconstruction the autografting method tested for the first time in a series of animal experiments by Bielschowsky and Unger (1917) has been gaining ground for a decade.

The introduction of the operating microscope and the development of the perineurial interfascicular suturing technique (Smith 1964, Michon and Masse 1964, Millesi, Ganglberger, and Berger 1967, Millesi 1968, 1969, 1972, Geldmacher 1969, Samii and Kahl 1972) have resulted in this method of grafting becoming a genuine step forward in the treatment of peripheral nerve injuries.

However, the disadvantages of this method should not be overlooked, especially whenever small gaps have to be closed. Autografting is impossible without losing another, albeit functionally less important donor nerve. Painful neuromas may develop on the proximal stump of the latter. There are always two suture lines required for the reconstruction of a nerve. Not infrequently, the distal suture line is constricted by scar tissue, which may enforce another resection and anastomosis later. If the size of the graft is insufficient its shrinking will generate tension which acts on the nerve. Moreover, the normal process of Wallerian degeneration and restitution will be upset because the formation of new blood vessels is insufficient to supply the graft (Sanders 1954). After autografting the speed of axon growth is 2 mm per day, whereas it is 3.5 mm per day after a simple end-to-end suture (Sanders and Young 1942). Both methods of operation will result in the return of motor function to about the same incomplete degree. After autografting, sensory recovery is slower and less complete (Krücke 1974).

In spite of these disadvantages, there is at present no alternative to autografting for bridging large gap distances. End-to-end suturing will probably hold its own for closing less extensive nerve defects and in some other isolated cases. There was, however, no answer to the question, what is the exact maximum length of a defect which can be safely repaired by an end-to-end suture without the use of any "manipulative" measures and without risking stretch injuries to the nerve? In other words, from what gap size upward is autografting indicated?

B. The Problem

It is the object of this paper to establish the limit of tolerable elongation beyond which severe injuries to the parenchyma will occur, impairing the regeneration of nerve tissue as well as the return of function after a simple circular suture. We intend to establish anew the critical resection length and critical gap distance pertaining to end-to-end sutures and to express their size as a percentage of the total nerve length. Critical resection length may either refer to a section to be resected from a still-continuous nerve (*e.g.*, a tumor), or to a loss of substance including that caused by freshening of stumps, after a traumatic lesion. The retraction of nerve ends is not taken into account in this case, whereas the dimension of critical gap distance always includes the size of the lesion as well as the extent of retraction which is present before initial debridement after a trauma.

To solve our clinical problem, therefore, we have to analyze the morphological changes taking place in a chronically stretched nerve in relation to the degree of strain applied. Furthermore, we have to collect data on the following subjects:

1. Mechanical properties of nerves.
2. Mechanical resistance and behaviour under strain of the tissues involved.
3. Nature and extent of the nerve lesions.
4. Ascent of the injury in the proximal portion of the nerve.
5. Individual variations in the consequences of stretching.
6. History of the degeneration and regeneration of the parenchyma.
7. Impairment of the neural vascular network and of the nutrient supply.
8. Retrograde cell reactions in the anterior columns of the spinal cord and in the spinal ganglia.

Additional data concerning

9. types and extent of muscular affection, and
10. clinical features

may be obtained by performing tensile tests on intact nerves.

Many experiments have been made to establish the fate of nerves subjected to brief acute stretching (Valentin 1864, 1881, Schleich 1871,

Verneuil 1876, Vogt 1877, Marcus and Wiet 1881, Prevost 1881, Scheving 1881, Witkowski 1881, Stintzing 1883, Takimoto 1916, Denny-
Brown and Doherty 1945, Schneider 1952, Haftek 1970). Histologically, the findings were fascicular oedema, hyperaemia, haemorrhages
in the epineurium and perineurium, rupture of the connective tissue
lamellae and discontinuity, with degeneration of nerve fibres which
regenerated later. These anatomical changes were related to motor,
sensory, and vegetative dysfunctions. Generally, no data concerning
tractive force or strain were given, and the nerve was stretched either
manually or by means of weights after surgical exposure.

The latest studies dealing with the critical degree of strain beyond
which the nerve will be injured were made by Highet and Sanders
(1943), Denny-Brown and Doherty (1945), Liu, Benda, and Lewey
(1948), Hoen and Brackett (1956), Sunderland and Bradley
(1961). The findings produced by these experiments vary because of
differences in measuring techniques and in the conditions of the
experiments, and also because of variations in morphological changes
which are due to differences in the species and nerve material
analyzed as well as to the age of the subject.

Liu, Benda, and Lewey (1948), Sunderland and Bradley (1961), and Sunderland (1972) used human nerves excised up to 12 hours after death. Studying the
mechanical behaviour of dead nerves and their tissues under tensile stress is a
clinically unreal and inadequate procedure. Vital reactions of nerves to permanent
and even to low tensile loads can be properly registered and charted only by
experiments on living subjects.

Highet and Sanders (1943), Denny-Brown and Doherty (1945), Hoen and
Brackett (1956) elongated the nerves of live animals. Denny-Brown and Doherty
(1945) stretched the sciatic nerves of cats after exposure by elongating a nerve
segment briefly with their fingers. This procedure, however, furnishes no data
concerning the magnitude of deformative force and stress. Unlike the case of a
nerve sutured end-to-end under tension, in which the tractive force acts towards
the suture line and tension spreads along the entire nerve, the direction of pull is
reversed in this case, and only a limited section of the nerve is subjected to
tension.

Highet and Sanders (1943) resected a certain portion of the common peroneal
nerve in dogs and reunited the two stumps with the knee fixed in a flexed position.
After 2 weeks, the nerve was either fully stretched by total removal of the
immobilization, or it was extended step by step in a turnbuckle cast. The experimental findings thus produced do not seem very helpful. Out of a total of seven
animal subjects, no more than two were reported to have their central nerve
stumps elongated by 6%, which was apparently tolerated. Histologically however, the suture lines had separated in both these cases and had been bridged by
longitudinal connective tissue.

Hoen and Brackett (1956) severed the sciatic nerves of dogs at various
distances distal to the femoral trochanter or the ischial tuberosity, suturing the
proximal end of the nerve to the tibia under extreme flexion of the knee. They
stretched the nerve by gradual extension of the extremity and by displacing the

fixation of the nerve stump caudally along the shinbone, leaving the distal segment of the nerve entirely out of consideration. Traction acted exclusively on the central segment of the nerve. The actual amount of traction exerted was not determined. The nerve was stretched and extended in stages. The exact rate of extension is difficult to determine because of the development of neuromas whose dimensions and development histories varied from one individual to another. Moreover, under everyday circumstances all central stump neuromas will always be resected completely. In addition to this, the parenchyma is changed because of the neuroma being injected with alcohol to alleviate the pain. Finally, it is nearly impossible to differentiate between damage caused by neurotomy and damage caused by strain.

C. Material and Methods

I. Selection of Appropriate Subjects

After some preliminary experiments on rabbits of 3 different breeds, albinos (average weight 2 kg), hare rabbits (4 kg), and German giant greys (6 kg), the latter breed proved to be best suited to our purpose. As far as our specific experiments were concerned, the length of their sciatic nerves was the major advantage of those giant rabbits. Measured from the spinal nerve roots to the terminal plate, the mean overall length of this nerve was 399 ± 15 mm.

II. Anatomy of the Sciatic Nerve in Rabbits

Unlike man, rabbits have 7 lumbar vertebrae and 7 lumbar spinal segments. Out of the 7 lumbar nerve roots, only roots 4–7 participate in the lumbar plexus. The sciatic nerve originates mainly in the 7th lumbar and 1st sacral nerve root and, to a lesser extent, in the 6th lumbar and 2nd and 3rd sacral roots.

The common peroneal nerve originates mainly from the 7th lumbar nerve, the tibial nerve and the motor branches of the sciatic nerve of the thigh originating from ansa lumbalis III. The saphenus minor nerve, which corresponds to the sural nerve in man, originates from the tibial nerve in the proximal part of the popliteal fossa.

A complete survey of the anatomy of the sciatic nerve in rabbits is given in the work of v. Ihering (1878), Krause (1884), and Gerhardt (1909).

III. Operative Technique

Our experiments were performed on 56 adult rabbits (30 male and 26 female) weighing on an average 5.96 ± 1.16 kg. We undermined no more than 10 mm of the sciatic nerve in the middle between the muscular branch to the semitendinosus, semimembranosus, and adductor magnus muscles and the bifurcation of the tibial and the common peroneal nerve. In this location, cylinders of various diameters were inserted and the nerves stretched by being looped around them. The cylinders were held in a position transversely to the sciatic nerves by being tacked to the adjacent connective and fascial tissue by means of Supramide sutures (Fig. 1). They remained in position *in vivo* until the animals were killed. We used stainless steel Sinox cylinders made by Schoeller Werk KG, D-5374, Hellenthal/ Eifel (length: 30 mm, wall thickness: 0.5 mm). While their radius varied from 1 to 5 mm, their weight remained low, ranging between 0.20 and 3.48 g, so that it seems safe to conclude that their weight alone could hardly compress the nerve to any injurious extent, even if they had not been retained in position. A cylinder implanted in this fashion does represent a bottleneck for the nerve to overcome, but there are quite a number of nerves which have to pass natural anatomical narrows.

We used five different cylinder circumferences (radius 1, 2, 3, 4, and 5 mm) to create five analogous degrees of strain, TG I, II, III, IV, and V, corresponding to a relative elongation of 2, 4, 6, 8, and 10% of the total nerve length. Strain was applied permanently over periods ranging from 1 day to a maximum of 35 weeks. Table 2 gives a survey of the numerical distribution of chronically extended sciatic nerves and the degree and duration of strain. As a rule, we elongated only the left sciatic nerve, the intact nerve on the other side being used for control purposes. We followed the same procedure in our studies of spinal ganglia, spinal cords, and muscles.

IV. Determination of the Critical Resection Length

The cylinder implantation method we used for stretching nerves permanently was developed for the purpose of studying the critical resection length in nerves. However, no actual resection of nerves took place. For our purpose, we assumed the resection of a nerve segment whose length corresponded exactly to the loop around the cylinder. As we were using 5 different cylinder circumferences, we had to analyze 5 different resection lengths as well as the corresponding elongations caused by an assumed end-to-end suture performed to close fictitious gaps. We assumed this fictitious neurorrhaphy to be located at the crossing of the distal and proximal parts of the loop. Analogous to the restoration of continuity which occurs after direct suture of a severed nerve, the continuity of the nerve between the proximal and the distal segment was preserved at the crossing of the two loop sectors (Fig. 2 a, b). Fig. 3 shows the defect sizes and the equivalent elongations of all 5 theoretical resection lengths in a dimensionally uniform system. These were the defects which would have to be overcome in order to achieve a restoration of continuity.

In absolute figures, the lengths of the segments theoretically resected from the rabbits' sciatic nerves were 6.28 mm (r_1 *); 12.57 mm (r_2); 18.85 mm (r_3); 25.13 mm (r_4); 31.42 mm (r_5). Related to the overall length of the sciatic nerve (319.0 ± 11.9 mm), they were equivalent to 1.97% ($\sim$ 2%); 3.94% ($\sim$ 4%); 5.91% ($\sim$ 6%); 7.88% ($\sim$ 8%); 9.85% ($\sim$ 10%) (see Table 3). The same significance was attributed to resection length, the size of the corresponding nerve gap in mm, and the tensile stress acting on a nerve with an

---

* r_1 = 1 mm cylinder radius = TG I.

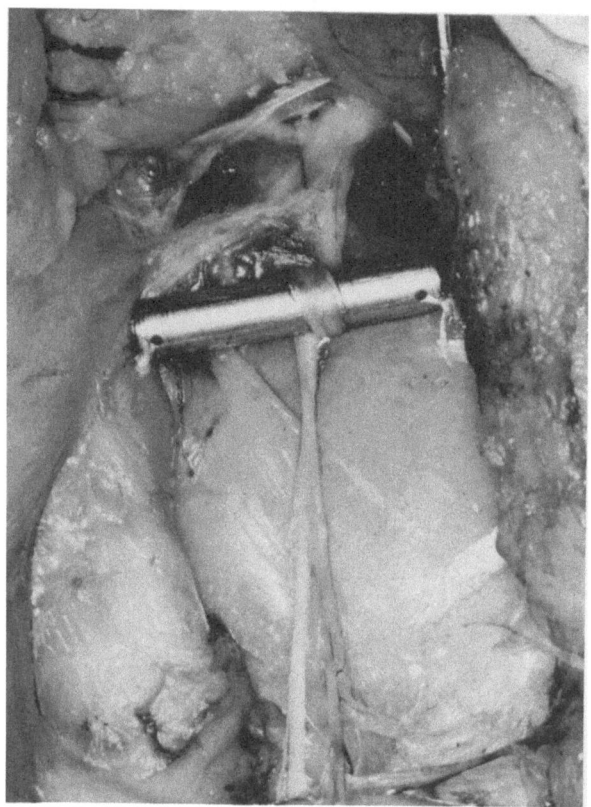

Fig. 1. Site of the operation and implanted cylinder (TG IV, r = 4 mm)

Table 2. *Breakdown of 56 Sciatic Nerves Into Degrees and Periods of Strain (TG = chronic degree of strain, d = day, w = week)*

TG	1d	2d	3d	4d	1w	2w	3w	4w	6w	8w	13w	30w	35w
I [r - 1mm]		1	1	1	3	1	1	1	2		1		
II [r - 2mm]	1	1		1	1	1	2	2	1		1		1
III [r - 3mm]		1		1	1	1	1	2		1	2		
I V [r - 4mm]	1	1	2	1	3	1		1		1	3		
V [r - 5mm]	1	1		1	1	1				1	1	1	

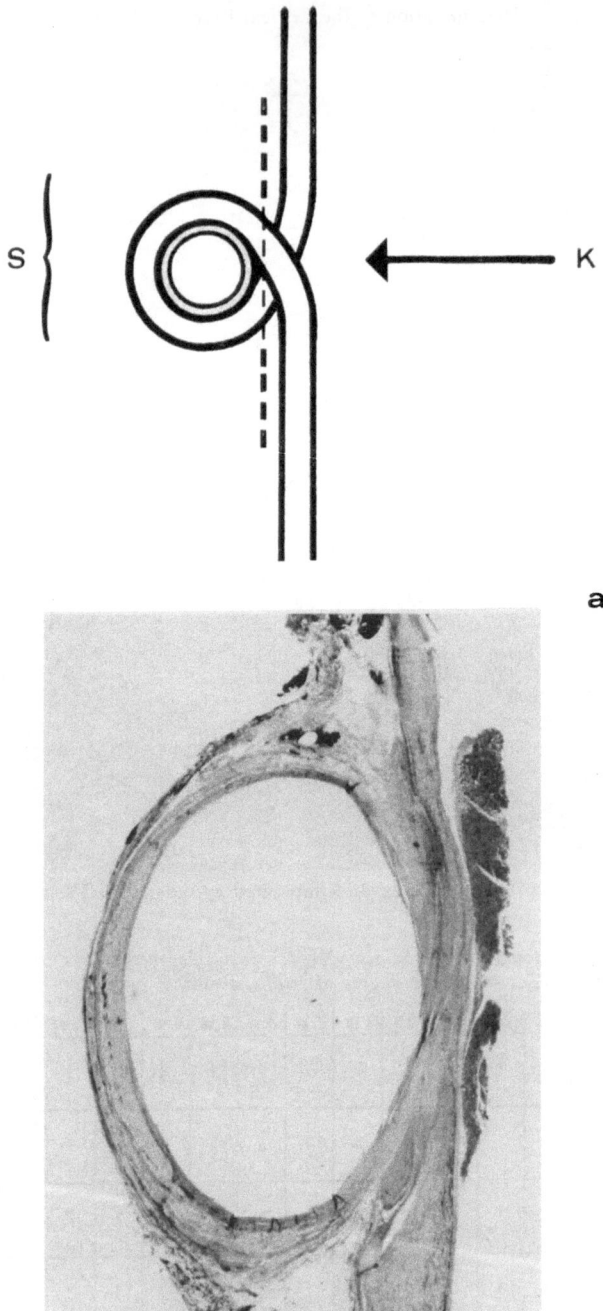

a

b

Fig. 2. Simulated resection length and suture of the sciatic nerve a) schematically,
b) morphologically (TG IV. Goldner. Magn. ×1.6). *S* nerve loop around the
cylinder = theoretical resection length, *K* crossing point of nerve ends in the
loop = site of the simulated suture

end-to-end suture bridging a defect. Our assumed resection lengths produced mechanical stresses in the rabbits' sciatic nerves which amounted to 0.028 (r_1), 0.056 (r_2), 0.083 (r_3), 0.111 (r_4), and 0.139 kp/mm² (r_5) (Table 3). The stresses acting on the stretched

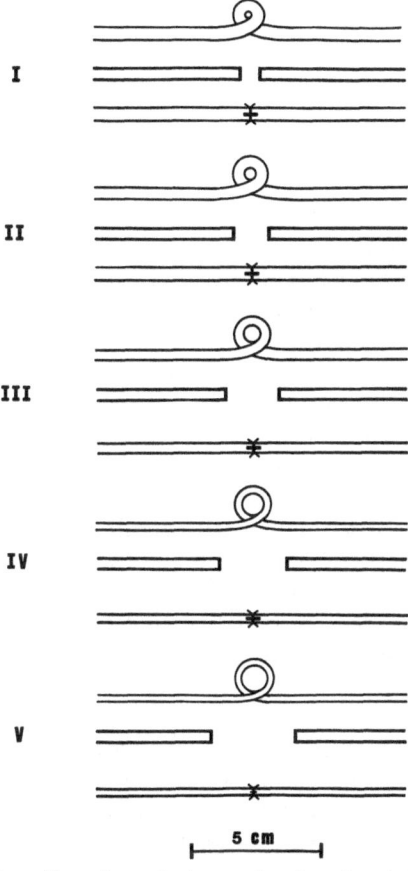

I

II

III

IV

V

|— 5 cm —|

Fig. 3. Plot comparing all 5 theoretical resection lengths (*I, II, III, IV, V*, top), their corresponding actual resection lengths (middle), and elongations caused by bridging the gap by end-to-end suturing (bottom)

nerves were computed according to Hooke's Law and confirmed by a parallel experiment (*cf.*, Chapter B/V, D/I).

Unlike actual nerve resections involving end-to-end tension sutures our experimental method excluded any possibility of being misled in assessing the histological situation by any processes of degeneration and regeneration which a neurotomy would have entailed. We were, therefore, in a position to concentrate exclusively on stretch injuries to the nerves, continuously analyzing their occurrence, their history, and their repair. Moreover, we established correlations between the strains and stresses acting on the nerves.

The initial strain and stress gradient occurring on the implantation of the cylinder were virtually equivalent to those occurring during the repair of a defect by a direct end-to-end suture between two nerve stumps, as was the attendant chronic nerve elongation. Similarly, the longitudinal traction acting towards the cylinder, or rather towards the theoretical suture, was comparable to the real situation. The stress originating at this point spreads uniformly throughout the entire nerve, centrally as well as peripherally.

V. Identification of Physical Parameters

It was necessary to determine exactly all physical factors so as to be able to gauge the relationship between stretch injuries to a peripheral nerve and the degree of strain, tractive force, and stress intensity.

According to the methods described above, a tractive force was applied to the nerve by means of an implanted cylinder. The circumference of each cylinder $(2\,r\,\pi)$ corresponds to the added length of the nerve Δl. Strain ε corresponds to the quotient of Δl and the original nerve length l, ranging from 2–10% (Table 3). The value used for l was not the absolute mean overall length of the sciatic nerve $(399 \pm 15$ mm) but 319.0 ± 11.9 mm: We subtracted from the former figure the length of the nerve segment in the distal half of the foot which consists of marked terminal ramifications. Given a foot length of 156 ± 19 mm, the length of this segment was approximately 80 mm.

To determine tractive force (K) and mechanical stress (σ) we ran a parallel experiment in the course of which we drew up the tractive force- and stress-strain diagrams of 12 normal, freshly resected sciatic nerves, each of which was taken from a different animal. We used the following apparatus for measuring the elongation of these nerves: The proximal end of each sciatic nerve was fixed firmly to a tripod. Its length (l) was measured under no load. Increasing the load or, rather, the tractive force acting on the nerve by 65 p* at each step, we used an optical measuring system to measure the added length (Δl), from which we computed the corresponding strain $\left(\varepsilon = \dfrac{\Delta l}{l}\right)$

We removed the load repeatedly to see if there was any remaining deformation. The load on the nerve was increased until the nerve

---

* p = pond (unit of weight). 1 p = 0.00981 N (Newton).

ruptured. Nerves were continuously sprayed with physiological saline while the measurements were being made to prevent desiccation.

Table 3. *Physical Results of Ex Corpore Elongation Experiments and Data of In Vivo Experiments (l = nerve length; F = nerve cross-section; E = Young's modulus; ε = strain; K = tractive force; K_z = breaking force; σ = stress; $σ_B$ = tensile strength; Δl = added length)*

ex corpore

l [mm]	F [mm²]	E [1] $\left[\dfrac{kp}{mm^2}\right]$	$ε$ [2] $= \dfrac{Δl}{l}$	$ε$ [2] %	K_z [kp]	$σ_B$ $\left[\dfrac{kp}{mm^2}\right]$
102,0 — 194,5	5,70 $\pm$0,32	1,41 $\pm$0,14	0,113 $\pm$0,029	11,3 $\pm$2,9	1,48 $\pm$0,22	0,246 $\pm$0,034

in vivo

l [mm]	cylinder radius [mm]	weight [p]	$2r\,π$ $= Δl$ [mm]	$ε$ $= \dfrac{Δl}{l}$	$ε$ %	K [kp]	$σ$ $\left[\dfrac{kp}{mm^2}\right]$
$\pm$ 319,0 $\pm$ 11,9	1	0,20	6,28	0,0197	1,97	0,158	0,028
	2	1,26	12,57	0,0394	3,94	0,317	0,056
	3	2,05	18,85	0,0591	5,91	0,475	0,083
	4	2,79	25,13	0,0788	7,88	0,633	0,111
	5	3,48	31,42	0,0985	9,85	0,792	0,139

[1] Compare: E in muscles = 0.001–0.1 approx. (Brecht 1967).
[2] Elongation before breaking = maximum elongation.

The stress (σ) generated in the elongated nerve was estimated from $σ = \dfrac{K}{F}$, with F representing the nerve diameter. We calculated the average diameter of 16 normal sciatic nerves which had been removed completely by dividing volume by nerve length, the mean result being 5.70 ± 0.32 mm². The volume of each sciatic nerve was determined by measuring its fluid displacement by means of a pyknometer.

We used all 12 tractive force- and stress-strain curves drawn up for each sciatic nerve to compute maps from which to read the tractive forces and mechanical stresses corresponding to the various degrees of strain applied in our experiment on live animals (Fig. 6 a, b). The two physical parameters can be computed even more exactly by applying Hooke's Law $\left(\Delta\ l = \dfrac{l \times K,}{F \times E} \right)$ with $K = \dfrac{\Delta l}{l} \times E \times F$ and $\sigma = \dfrac{K}{F} = \dfrac{\Delta l}{l} \times E$. Therefore, at each degree of strain (1, 2, 3, 4, and 5 mm cylinder radius) the tractive force varied between 0.158 and 0.792 kp, the stress values ranging between 0.028 and 0.139 kp/mm^2 (Table 3).

In the course of our *ex corpore* strain tests we were able to gain information about yield point, flow limit, maximum elongation, tensile strength, breaking point and breaking force as well. Young's modulus was also determined by way of Hooke's Law: $E = \dfrac{l \times K}{\Delta l \times F}$

VI. Clinical Studies

As far as the differences in the experimental survival periods of the animals would allow, we recorded our clinical findings on the following points at 2-day intervals:

a) Decubitus

In addition to the size of the trophic ulcers we recorded the time elapsed before their occurrence as well as the time required for complete healing.

b) Perception of Pain

Practically speaking, reliable data on superficial sensation could be gained only by observing the quality of pain. We judged the amount of pain perceived by the defensive movements of the shank and especially by dorsal and plantar flexion, which meant that motor power had to be either completely normal or only partly impaired.

c) Motor Reactions

Provocative tests, during which the animals were dropped from a random height, showed a reflex dorsal flexion of the foot and a splaying of the phalanges in all lower extremities which were either intact or showed only slight motor defects, whereas paralyzed extremities continued to hang down flaccidly. Moreover, we used painful stimuli to cause movements of the affected extremity.

d) Atrophy

Pendl (1963) stated that it is more reliable to gauge atrophy macroscopically by muscle weight rather than by measuring the circumference of an extremity. The azygous soleus muscle was best suited to this purpose, and we excised a coherent segment of it over a length of 8.5 cm, the area of maximum circumference always being in the centre of the segment excised. To preclude any possible errors being caused by differences in muscle weight due to perfusion we recorded the difference between the intact soleus muscle on one side and the pathological muscle on the other in %.

VII. Histological Studies

Under Nembutal anaesthesia the laboratory animals were perfused trans-cardially via the ascending aorta with Periston heated to body temperature, followed by a perfusion with 10% acid-free formalin. Immediately after perfusion, we excised both sciatic nerves, both soleus muscles, the lumbo-sacral spinal cord together with its adjacent spinal roots, ganglia and the nerves on both sides for histological examination. The sciatic nerve was excised from its point of exit through the greater sciatic notch to the ankle joint.

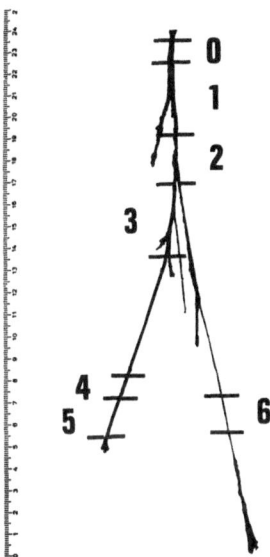

Fig. 4. Survey of numbered and histologically analyzed nerve segments. Proximal nerve end: Greater sciatic notch. Distal end: Ankle joint region. Segments 0–2 Nerve trunk, 2 Cylinder region, 3–5 Tibial nerve, 6 Peroneal nerve

With all its branches, it was spread out free of tension, its dimensions were measured, and its shape and macroscopic changes were either photographed or documented by drawings. The sciatic as well as the peroneal and the tibial nerve after their bifurcation were dissected into segments to produce histological longitudinal and cross-sections. All segments were numbered continuously from proximal to distal (Fig. 4). In addition to incorporating the loop, segment 2 also contains a proximal and distal segment whose length varies with the circumference of the cylinder. All other segment were studied as well. The thickness of the paraffin section was 10 μ and that of the celloidon specimens was 15–20 μ. We used the following staining methods: Bodian, Klüver, Klüver-Barrera, Masson-Goldner, v. Gieson, Nissl, and HE.

In addition to this, the specimens taken from the belly of the soleus muscle were embedded in gelatine and stained with black and red Sudan.

The vascular system of 10 rabbits was subjected to a comparative analysis of stretched and normal sciatic nerves. Out of that number, the following were subjected to the various degrees of strain: TG I = 2, II = 1, III = 4, IV = 2, and V = 1. After 1–3 days of permanent nerve stretching, the vasa nervorum were identified by a perfusion of undiluted, twice-filtered Skriptol Indian ink made by G. Wagner. The ink was heated to body temperature and injected *intra vitam* into the ascending aorta. Before this perfusion, we used Periston (1000 ml, 37 °C) to flush the blood from the vascular system. Clamping the v. cava caudalis before ending the injection caused a brief increase of pressure in the venous and the capillary circulation system, so that even the terminal vascular regions were well filled with Skriptol. We did not use any drugs such as papaverin or heparin.

We then measured the ischaemic section of the stretched nerve, which had become identifiable macroscopically because it was either not stained at all or only imperfectly so.

After the usual preliminary treatment, we kept the perfused nerves for 1 week in oil of wintergreen for transparency so as to facilitate microscopic studies. After this, they were embedded in celloidon and cut into longitudinal sections of 200 μ thickness.

D. Results

Instead of giving a global survey we shall present each result individually, describing it in a separate chapter.

I. Mechanical Properties

a) Findings

Depending on the qualitative and quantitative composition of the tissue components there may be individual variations in the elastic behaviour of nerves. The strain curves of the sciatic nerves of 12 rabbits shown in Fig. 5 a, b demonstrate individual variations of this kind. Under the same tractive forces and stresses the amount of strain sustained by each nerve will vary more or less from the mean. These divergences in extensibility do not occur so much under initial loading but are most clearly marked when the nerve is subjected to higher tensile loading or stress. All individual linear curves show that strain and tractive force are proportional. The last entry on each curve represents the maximum load reached before a sciatic nerve ruptures. As tensile strength varies, the breaking point is bound to vary as well, the loads generally ranging from 0.59 to 1.90 kp but reaching 2.45 kp in one case. The following mean values have been established for our physical measurements: Breaking force (K_z) : 1.48 ± 0.22 kp; tensile strength (σ_B) : 0.246 ± 0.034 kp/mm²; maximum elongation (ε) 0.113 ± 0.029 in absolute figures or 11.3 ± 2.9%. Young's modulus was calculated at $E = 1.41$ ± 0.14 kp/mm² (see top of Table 3). Scatter bandwidths are described in detail in chapter E/I [*].

Fig. 6 a and b show mean curves and standard deviations of all tractive force-strain and stress-strain diagrams, respectively. We can see that, *in vivo*, our five degrees of strain have the following values:

TG [**]	ε (%)	K (kp) Mean value including standard deviation	σ (kp/mm²) Mean value including standard deviation
I	2	0.050–0.110–0.160	0.011–0.021–0.030
II	4	0.200–0.250–0.320	0.033–0.048–0.070
III	6	0.330–0.390–0.510	0.052–0.075–0.108
IV	8	0.450–0.540–0.650	0.074–0.101–0.131
V	10	0.750–0.930–1.110	0.130–0.158–0.169

[*] Measurements were evaluated statistically after Kohlrausch (1968).
[**] TG = chronic degree of strain (elongation).

2*

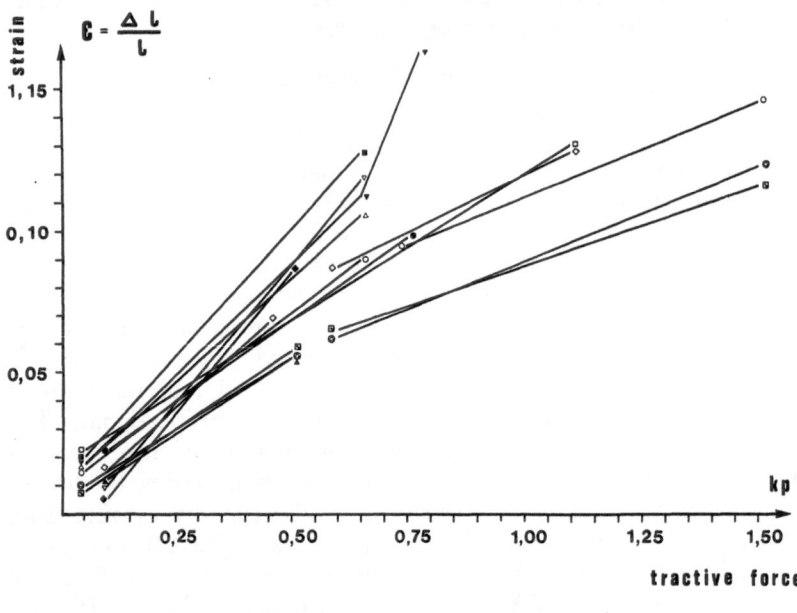

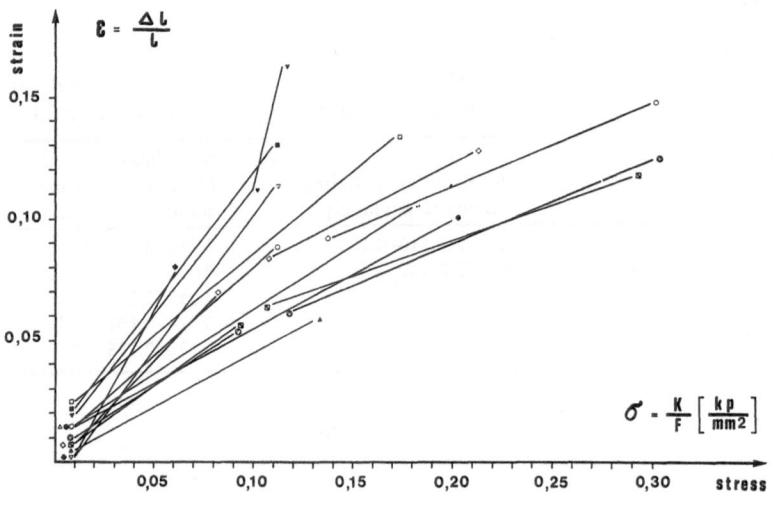

Fig. 5. Tractive force—strain diagram (a) and stress—strain diagram (b) of 12 sciatic nerves excised from different individuals. Approximated lines. Line approximation performed after Duschek (1963)

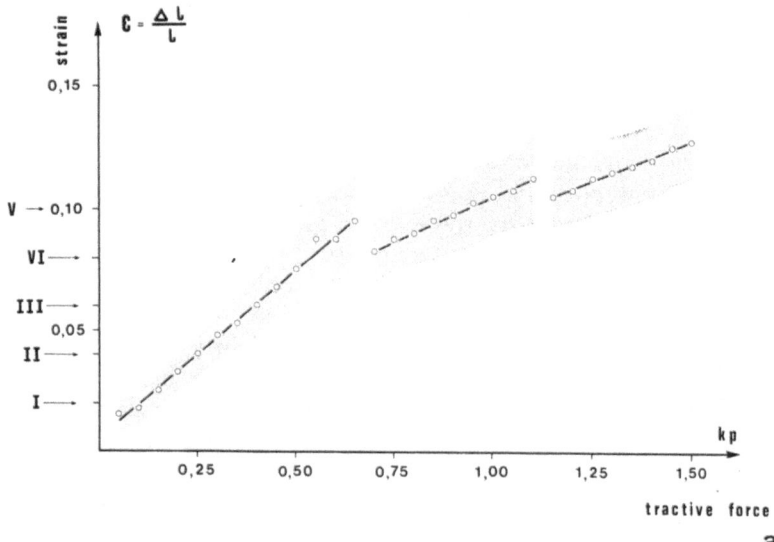

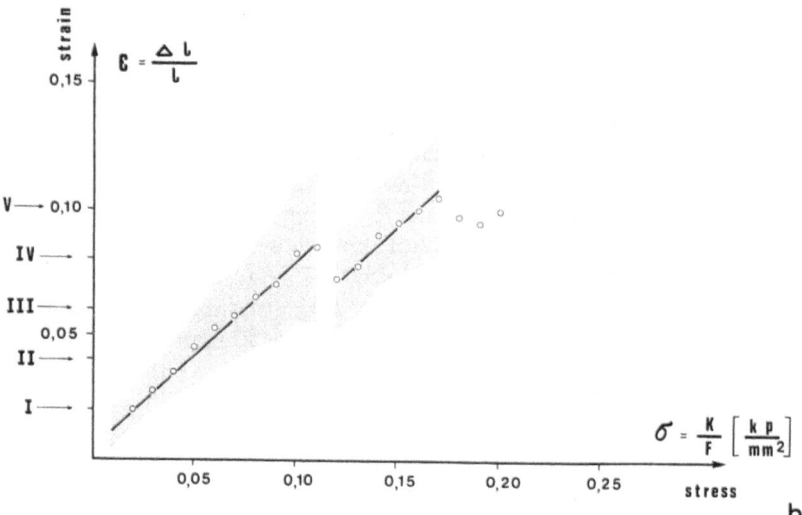

Fig. 6. Tractive force—strain diagram (a) and stress—strain diagram (b). Mean curve derived from the approximated lines of Fig. 5 a, b

There is a 15% difference in the tractive force figures and a 20% difference in the stress figures between those given above and those computed according to Hooke's Law (see bottom of Table 3), the latter being still within the standard deviation range.

Discontinuities in the mean value curves are caused by nerves breaking and ceasing to be measurable. Within our range of measurement, no major nerve deformation was observed after removing the load. Flow limit, yield point and breaking point, which are reached one after the other as the tractive force increases in stages of 0.065 kp and the stress increases in stages of 0.011 kp/mm^2, are all outside the curves shown in Fig. 5 a, b. There is only one instance where a nerve shows a distinct flow or yield point (▼ —— ▼). Before breaking, with the tractive force increased only slightly, this nerve showed an excessive increase in elongation, irreversible deformation, and semi-plastic behaviour. Curves begin to flatten out as the tractive force increases beyond 0.6 to 1.6 kp and the stress increases beyond 0.1–0.3 kp/mm^2. This indicates that a nerve, when subjected to any major load, will change its mechanical properties and therefore lose some of its stretching capacity. So we can conclude that the elastic limit and the proportional limit have already been transgressed, the latter being empirically very close to the former.

b) Discussion

As early as 1931, Nauck, in his studies on the mechanical and functional significance of nerve undulation, observed a certain variation in the extensibility of nerves. Differences in the tensile strength of human sciatic nerves are based not only on individual but also on racial factors (Tillaux as quoted by Blum 1878, Gillette 1880, Trombetta 1880, Symington 1882, Takimoto 1916). Sunderland and Bradley (1961), Hartung and Arnold (1973), found a considerable bandwidth of maximum loads, tensile strengths, maximum elongations, and points of mechanical failure in other human nerves (ulnar, median, and popliteal nerves as well as the spinal nerve roots).

Schneider (1952) even reported extensive variations in tensile strength between individual isolated fibres of the sciatic nerve in frogs. These variations even occurred among individuals of the same species, sex, and age group. However, he found sciatic nerves excised from one individual to be identical to a remarkable extent.

The mechanical resistance of nerves depends mainly on their connective tissue sheaths (Schneider 1952, et al.). Moreover, the connective tissue of a nerve is more elastic than the nerve itself.

As the nerve divides distally into a number of fascicles, the proportion of perineurial and interfascicular connective tissue increases. Yet there always remains a linear relationship between fascicle diameter and the thickness of the perineurium. As the relative proportion of connective tissue increases, the elastic quality of the peripheral nerve segments improves, while their tensile strength increases because of their inner plexus formations (Sunderland 1972). As the isolated nerve roots are not embedded in powerful connective tissue membranes, and as their individual fibres are running parallel to each other, they are sooner and more intensely affected by stretching (Sunderland and Bradley 1961).

While the macroscopic anatomical continuity of nerves remains intact throughout the quasilinear range of strain diagrams and up to their upper limit (Figs. 5 a, b, 6 a, b) this does not mean that the neurophysiological functions of the nerves have remained unaffected as well. The resistance of both the axons and their myelin sheaths to stress is much lower (Liu, Benda, and Lewey 1948). We will corroborate this statement by the results of our own investigations. We are therefore in a position to state that connective tissue sheaths will not protect the nerve parenchyma from the effects of stretching.

II. Clinical Observations

a) Findings

Decubitus: Trophic lesions occur most frequently in the region of the heel. There is no connection between the size and the development of these skin ulcers and the degree of stretching of the sciatic nerve. For instance, some of the extreme cases of ulceration recorded in TG I animals began after a mere 8 days, whereas TG V animals showed ulceration after 26 weeks. The same discrepancies occur in the progress of skin injuries as well as in their healing. However, the number of animals free from extensive trophic disturbances was remarkably high in the rabbits subjected to TG I and much lower in those animals which were subjected to higher degrees of strain.

During the initial stage, some cases will develop soft tissue oedema in their distal extremities (*cf.*, Neri 1909). As early as 1882, Quinquaud observed a case of enormous elephantiasis, while Stintzing (1883) reported joint swellings.

Perception of pain: 100% of all TG III–V cases showed analgesia on the first post-operative day. In 58% of all TG II cases, sensitivity to pain disappeared in the course of the first 5 days. Analgesia occurred in a mere 17% of all TG I cases, the onset being delayed by as much as 1 month in one case.

Motor reactions: As we judged the presence of algesia by the defensive movements of the shank and especially by dorsal and plantar flexion, our findings regarding nociperception also indicate the extent of mobility. Consequently, analgesia, as a rule, is accompanied by paralysis. We saw no indication of recovery from analgesia and paralysis, the sole exceptions being 3 TG II cases which we observed for 13 weeks. In one TG V case, the sensory and motor functions did not begin to return before the 27th week.

Atrophy: There is no correlation between the loss of weight of the soleus muscle and the extent to which the nerve is stretched (Fig. 7 a). The highest loss of weight in the soleus muscle was 67.6% recorded in the 6th week of TG II.

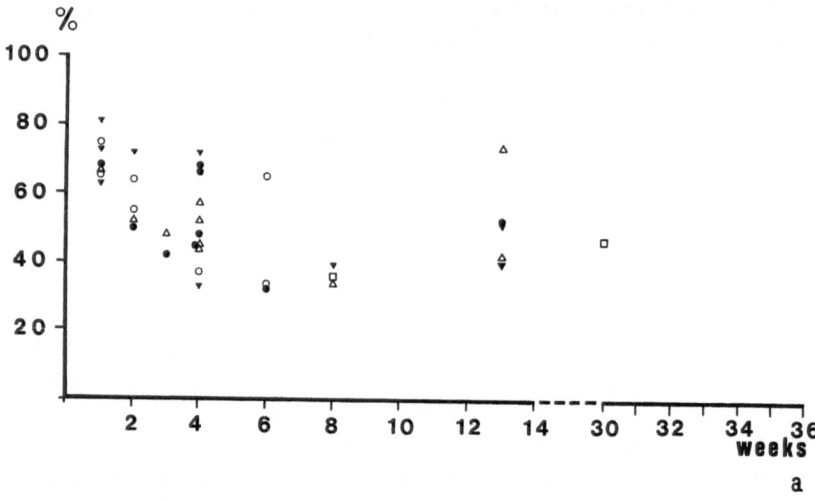

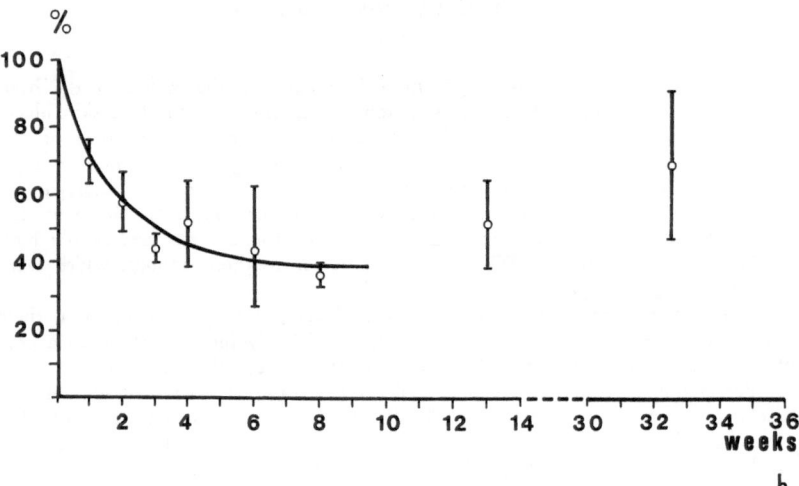

Fig. 7. Loss of weight in the soleus muscle under permanent sciatic nerve stretching. a) Individual values under TG I ○, II ●, III △, IV ▼, V □, b) Regression curve disregarding degrees of strain

The other maximum figures are: TG I, 67.2%, 6th week; TG III, 65.8%, 8th week; TG IV, 66.7%, 4th week; and TG V, 63.8%, 8th week. The curve on Fig. 7 b shows the regression of the mean weights of the soleus muscle. Initially, there is a steep drop which abates somewhat until finally, figures approximating 40% of the initial weight are shown for the 8th and 9th week, whereas the muscle weight seems to be increasing again in the 13th week.

b) Discussion

Neri (1909) found the functional lesions caused by stretching of the sciatic nerve for periods ranging from 40 hours to 4 days to be irreparable. After traction lasting 10, 15, and 24 hours, periods of 1, 2, and 3 months respectively were required to return to normal sensation and movement. Conrad (1876), Debove and Laborde (1881), and Scheving (1881) found that stretching the sciatic nerve briefly caused either a marked decrease or a complete disappearance of sensation, while movement was not affected at all. On the other hand, disturbances of movement were never found to occur unless accompanied by disturbances of sensation (Takimoto 1916). Functional changes were found to be dependent on tractive force, but the relationship was a relatively gradual one (Stintzing 1883, Takimoto 1916). It seemed that, as the tractive force increases, sensation is affected first and movement later.

As opposed to those findings, our experiments showed a continuous relationship between sensation and movement disturbances, independent of the degree of chronic strain acting on the sciatic nerve, the duration of the paresis being a better criterion of the seriousness of the stretch injury than its intensity. Stintzing (1883) was also unable to produce even a slight reduction of sensation without causing a paresis at the same time.

The loss of weight of the soleus muscle, which fluctuates widely and does not depend on the degree of strain applied, seems to be caused by individual characteristics. Ricker and Ellenbeck (1899) found individual variations in the loss of weight of the triceps surae muscle even after neurotomy. We may safely assume that under nerve elongation, too, the extent of atrophy in a muscle is determined mainly by factors specific to the individual. Moreover, in terms of weight the atrophy of muscles is influenced by the variations in the elastic properties of the individual sciatic nerves and by the quantitative differences in stretch injuries recorded even among cases of the same degree of strain.

The period of time required to reach the final stage of muscle weight loss agrees with the findings of Thulin and Carlsson (1969) concerning muscular atrophy caused by denervation after severing the anterior nerve roots, and those of Ricker and Ellenbeck (1899) concerning the effects of sciatic nerve section. However, the weight reduction figures produced by our experiment were less by 9 and 19%, respectively.

III. Macroscopic Findings

None of the degrees of strain applied ever resulted in a primary or a secondary interruption of the nerve due to ischaemic necrosis, either at the point of application of the tractive force or at the nerve roots, so that the continuity of the sciatic nerve was preserved from its origin in the cord to its terminal ramifications. Moreover, there was no evidence of peripheral branches being torn away from the nerve trunk or from the innervated organ.

Fig. 8 is a comparison between a normal sciatic nerve and a nerve changed by chronic stretching. Haemorrhages develop in the outer nerve sheaths. Their proximal and distal extent depends on the degree of strain. The haemorrhages produced by TG I in the cylinder region are only slight and are obviously due to the operation itself. These haemorrhages are absorbed by the 10th day, whereas those produced by the other degrees of strain can be observed beyond the second week. Moreover, ecchymoses occur where distal nerve branches enter the muscles. Extravasation caused by brief stretching disappears after one week (Vogt 1877, Stintzing 1883, Takimoto 1916).

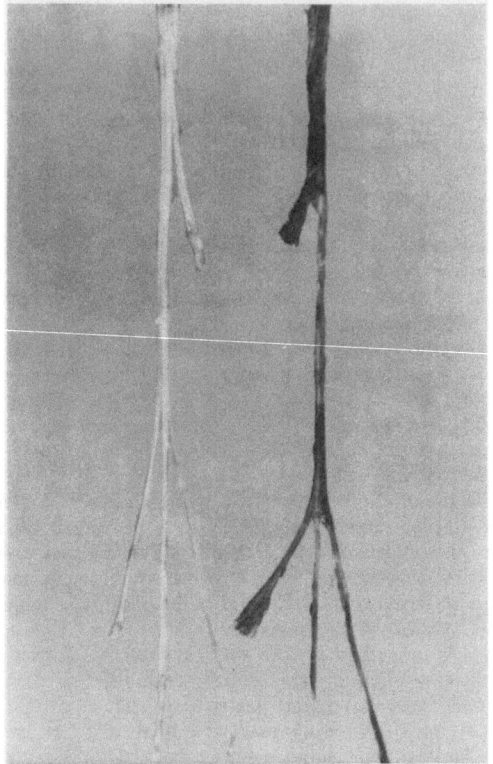

Fig. 8. Nerve stretched under TG V (right). 1st day. Showing superficial haemorrhages throughout. Left: Normal sciatic nerve

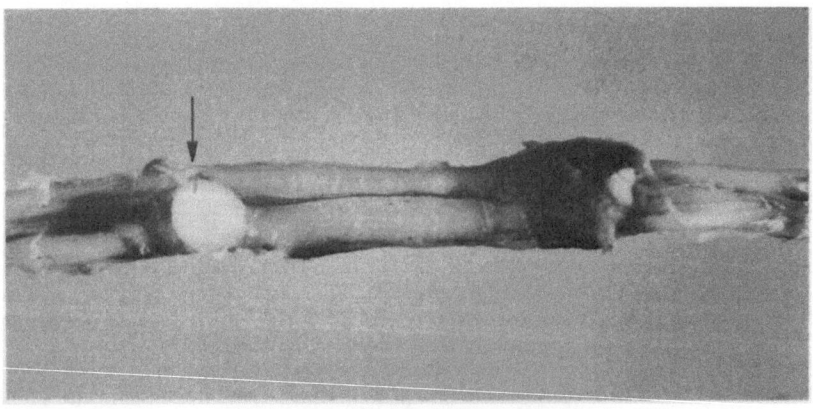

Fig. 9. Neural hernia. TG IV. 4th day

Moreover, nerves reduced in calibre are identified by dull, whitish, ischaemic patches and by their flabby consistency after haemorrhages have been absorbed. Some are marked by diffuse swellings caused by a proliferation of epineurial connective tissue. Takimoto (1916) reports circumscribed increases in thickness caused by transitory traction.

Extensive morphological changes were produced only by TG IV and V, where neural herniae occurred in 50% of all cases during the first week. These herniae, both acute and subacute, manifested themselves mainly in areas of increased stress. In 2 cases, their onset was observed during the operation, immediately after the cylinder was implanted. Six nerves were affected by solitary herniation. Only one nerve showed a multiple hernia (3). The largest hernia of nerve parenchyma recorded, measured 3.5 by 3.0 mm (Fig. 9).

IV. Histological Results

1. Sciatic Nerve

a) Findings: All degrees of strain caused morphological lesions in the chronically stretched sciatic nerves without reaching the elastic limit. The extent of a lesion depends on the resistance of the individual tissue components to mechanical loading. The following tissue components are named in the order of decreasing resistance: Epineurium, perineurium, endoneurium, blood vessels, axons, and myelin sheaths.

Even a low amount of strain will eliminate the natural undulation of the nervous as well as the fibrous components and distend the Schmidt-Lantermann incisures. From TG II onwards, both the axons and the endoneurial tissue fibres are elongated initially. Under TG I, stretching becomes evident only gradually, as it is caused not so much by the original strain as by additional dynamic tensile loading of the sciatic nerve, the extent of which depends on the range of motion of the extremity. Unlike the distal branches, the proximal motor ramifications of the sciatic nerve branching off into the thigh muscles are not affected by stretching. Their normal undulation is preserved or even compressed lengthwise.

The very first changes to become evident in the parenchyma occur in the myelin sheaths. Swellings occur in the areas adjacent to Ranvier's nodes (Fig. 10), followed by a retraction of the myelin substance. The uniform honeycomb longitudinal structure of the myelin layer is destroyed, as is its typical wheel-spoke cross-section. Under TG I, the latent period before the actual onset of demyelination may range from 3–7 days, whereas degeneration is immediate in TG II–V and progresses rapidly in those segments which are under high stress.

All axons which are under increased stress are stretched thin, and their normal spindle-shaped and sometimes bamboo-like segmentation disappears (Fig. 11 a, b).

Some axons will rupture if the nerve is elongated by a mere 4% (TG II) (Fig. 12). In these cases, as distinct from those of neurotomy, nerve discontinuity is not limited to a particular level but spread widely over a large number of places. The number of ruptured nerve fibres increases with the degree of strain, and axons rupture at increasing proximal and distal distances from the cylinder region. Of

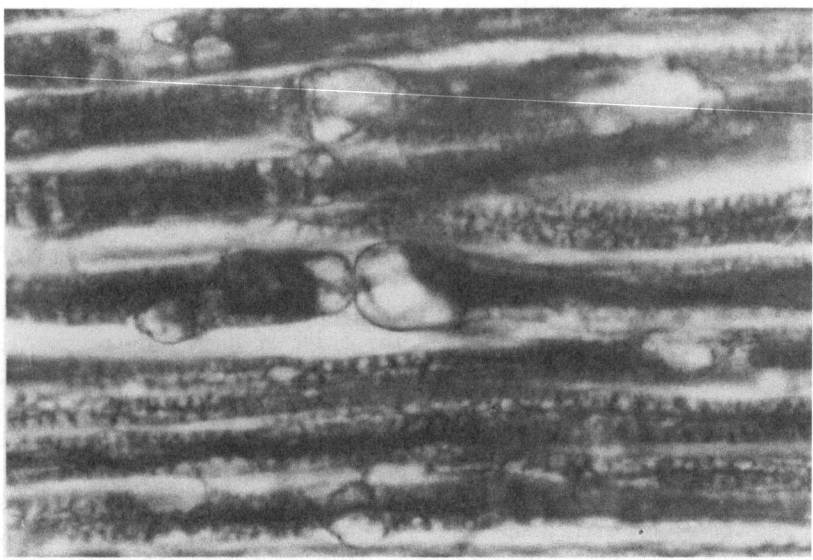

Fig. 10. Position of subtraction and incipient discontinuity of myelin sheaths in the region of Ranvier's nodes. TG II. 1st day. NS * 1. Goldner. Magn. ×256

the overstretched and broken axons, only spiral, serpentine, or glomerular fragments are left (Fig. 13). There are single as well as multiple ruptures. As a rule, in neural herniae produced by TG IV and V all axons are ruptured. In general, remnants of ruptured axons are only rarely evident later than the end of the 2nd week of stretching (Fig. 14).

Additional injuries to the nerve parenchyma are caused by traction acting on the vasa nervorum. In addition to ischaemia, the stretched nerve suffers from acute or subacute haemorrhage due to angiorrhexis, and eventually, obstructive changes will occur in the vascular supply of the nerve. Most haemorrhages occur subepineurially or subperineurially, and from TG II onwards they are found

---

* NS = nerve segment (cf. Fig. 4).

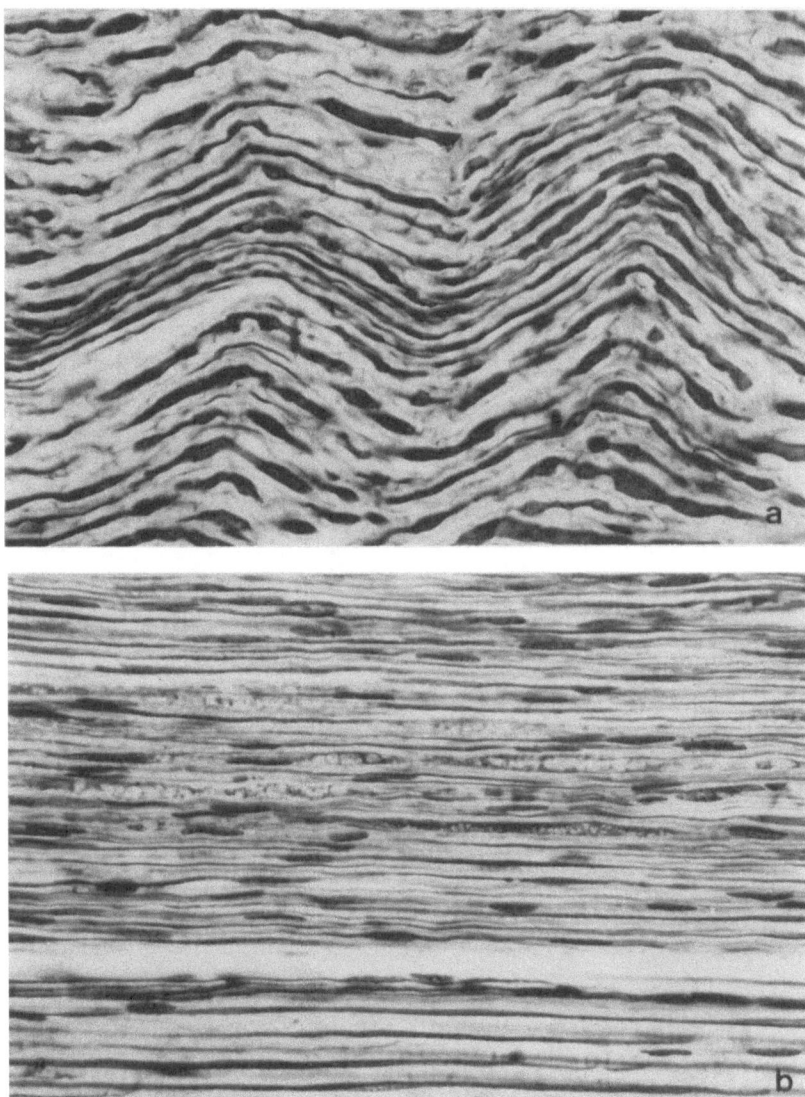

Fig. 11. a) Undulation of normal nerve fibres. Occasional bamboo-like structure of axons. Bodian. Magn. ×128. b) Stretched thin axons. TG V. 4th day. NS 5. Bodian. Magn. ×128

proximally and distally (Fig. 15). From the third week onwards, all histological evidence of extravasation disappears, and scar tissue resulting from its organization is reduced to a minimum. In some instances of TG II–V, the thickness of the tunica intima fluctuated

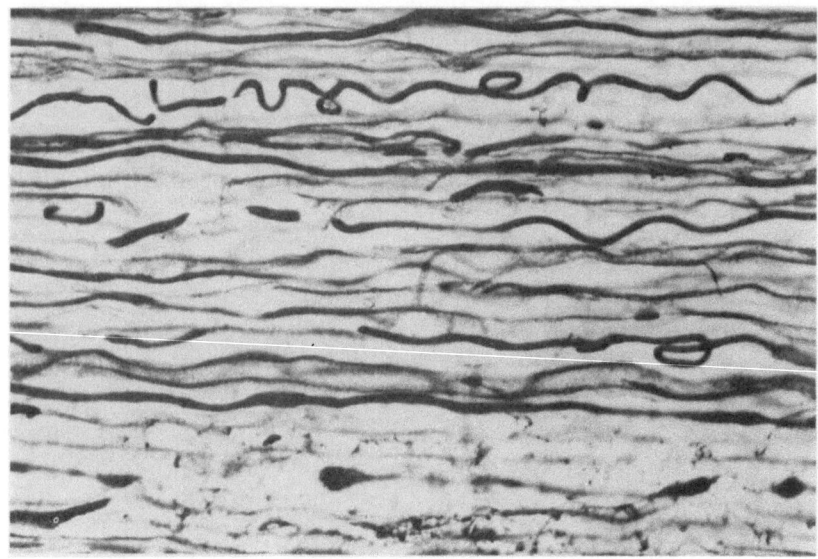

Fig. 12. Single and multiple axon ruptures. TG II. 1st week. NS 3. Bodian.
Magn. ×160

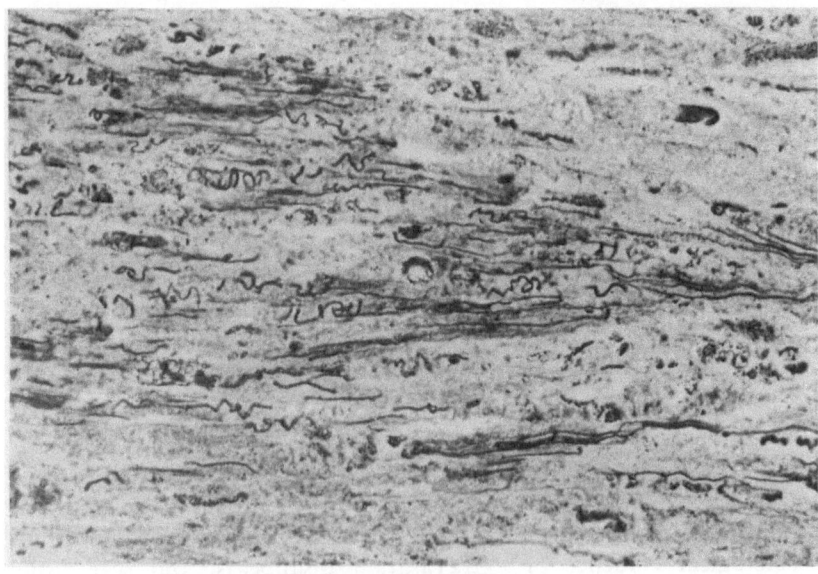

Fig. 13. Corkscrew-shaped fragments of ruptured axons. TG V. 1st week. NS 1.
Bodian. Magn. ×100

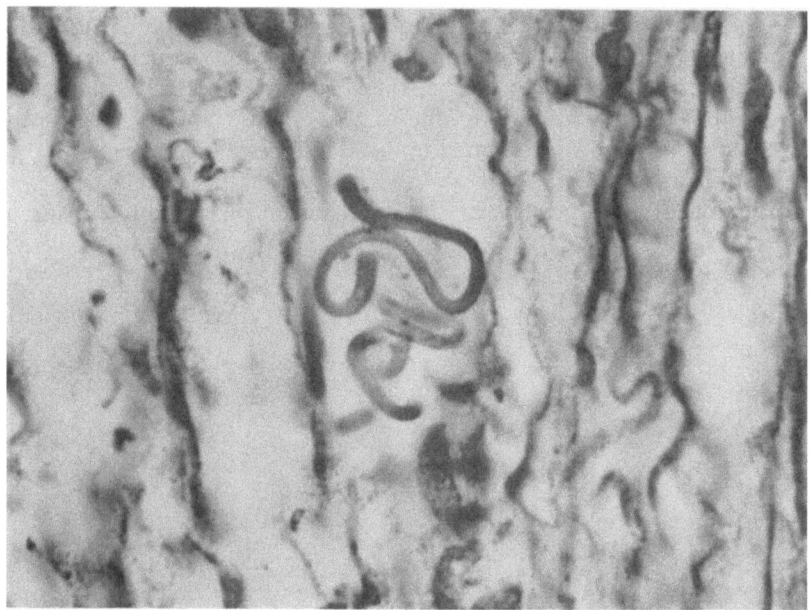

Fig. 14. Loop-shaped remnant of an axon. TG III. 4th week. NS 2. Bodian.
Magn. ×256

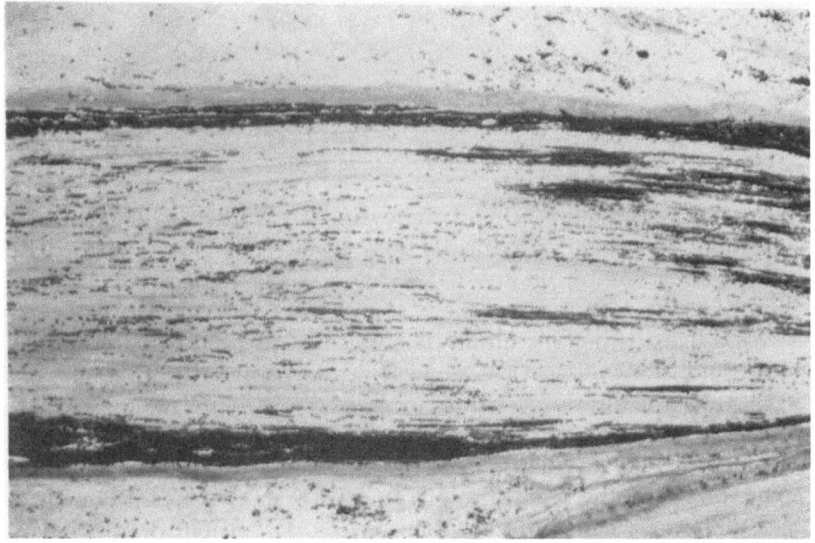

Fig. 15. Sites of haemorrhages of mainly subperineurial and slight intraneural
extent. TG V. 1st week. NS 5. Goldner. Magn. ×25.6

widely from the 6th week onwards, due to proliferation of the endothelium. Although the diameter of the blood vessels was thus constricted to a varying degree, there were only a few instances of occlusion which were mainly due to thrombosis. Nearly all cases of venous congestion were located in distal nerve segments (Fig. 16).

Permanent TG I strain on the nerve sheaths merely led to a reduction of the thickness of the perineurium on the convex side of

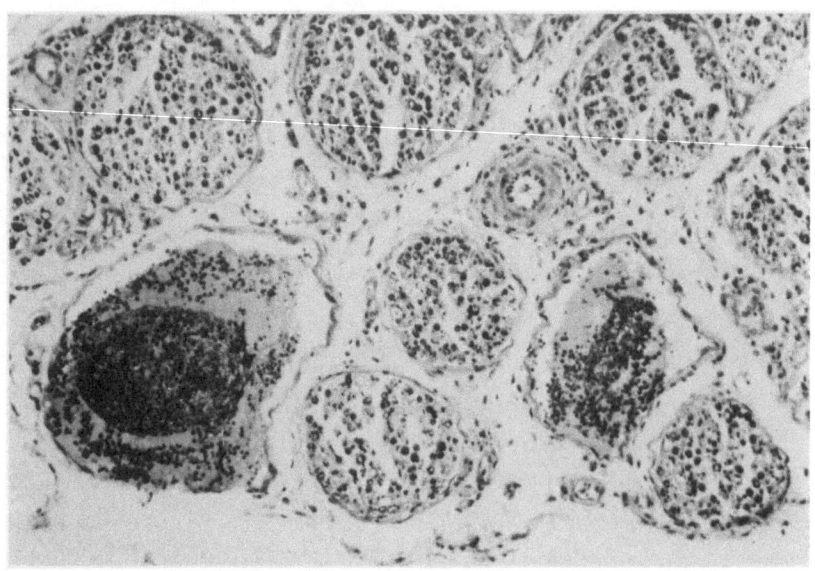

Fig. 16. Stasis in endoneurial veins accompanied by dissociation of the inner wall. Fascicles contain some myelinated nerve fibres still intact. TG III. 2nd week. NS 4. Goldner. Magn. ×40

the nerve loop wound around the cylinder. Under TG II, the same condition was found proximally and distally, obviously caused by uneven stress acting on the nerve and on the parenchyma as well (Fig. 17 a, b). This unevenness seems to disappear as strain increases; at least, there is no morphological evidence of it. Individual fibres of the endoneurial, epineurial and perineurial connective tissues begin to rupture as strain increases. We found the most severe complication to be a rupture of both epineurium and perineurium accompanied by a prolapse of the parenchyma, which occurred under elongations ranging from 8 to 10% (TG IV and V, Figs. 18 and 19). Neural herniae can be either macroscopically visible or microscopically small, but they are always external (Fig. 18). Smaller herniae only involve a partial rupture of the connective tissue

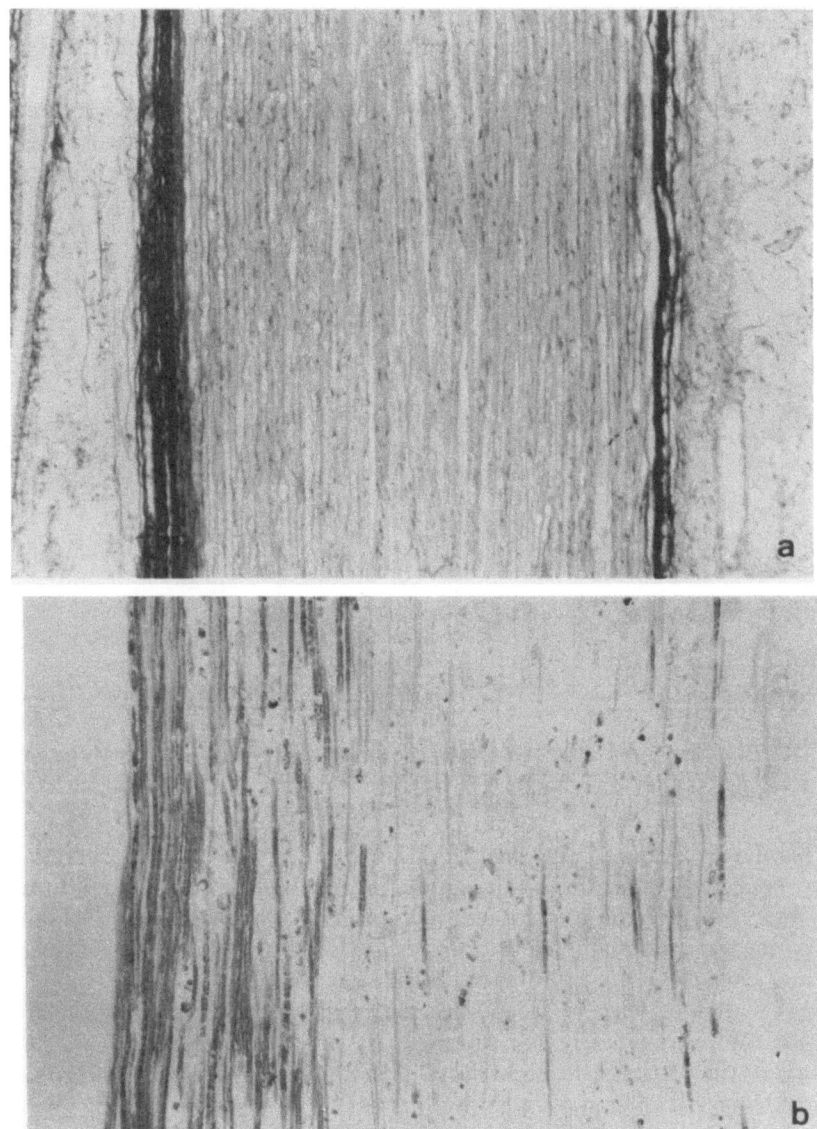

Fig. 17. Mainly unilateral stretch effects on the convex side. a) Narrowing of the integumentum externum. TG II. 1st week. NS 3. Van Gieson. Magn. ×25.6. b) Increased disintegration of parenchyma. TG I. 6th week. NS 2 proximal to the simulated suture. Klüver. Magn. ×40

sheath (Fig. 20). Herniations occur exclusively in the main fascicles of the sciatic nerve trunk and are always accompanied by haemorrhages at the hernial orifice. The hernial contents consist of completely destroyed nerve tissue. Only in microscopically small herniae, a few small-calibre nerve fibres located well away from the hernial orifice may survive intact. In the

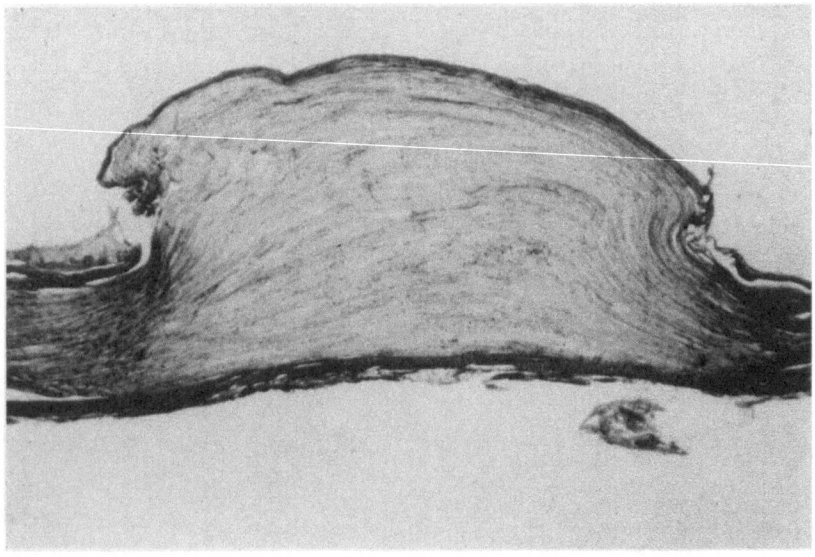

Fig. 18. Longitudinal section of a nerve hernia. Epineurium and perineurium totally ruptured at the left side of the hernial orifice. TG V. 1st week. NS 2. Van Gieson. Magn. ×12.8

herniated segments, the disintegration of the parenchyma progresses more quickly than the Wallerian degeneration elsewhere. We did not observe any of the pseudo-neuromas which form around the prolapse of the parenchyma after brief stretching of the nerve (Denny-Brown and Doherty 1945, Liu, Benda, and Lewey 1948).

Wallerian degeneration even affects those nerve fibres which are not injured primarily by rupture. Its onset occurs somewhere between the first and the eighth day after the commencement of chronic stretching. The higher the strain, the earlier the process of disintegration becomes manifest. It depends on the intraneural level of stress, which decreases proximally and distally. Initially regressive phenomena are more numerous in areas of high stress, whereas in areas of low stress degeneration is delayed and affects a lesser proportion of the nerve fibres. Initially, we therefore have apparently intact nerve fibres as well as nerve fibres in the initial or later stages of

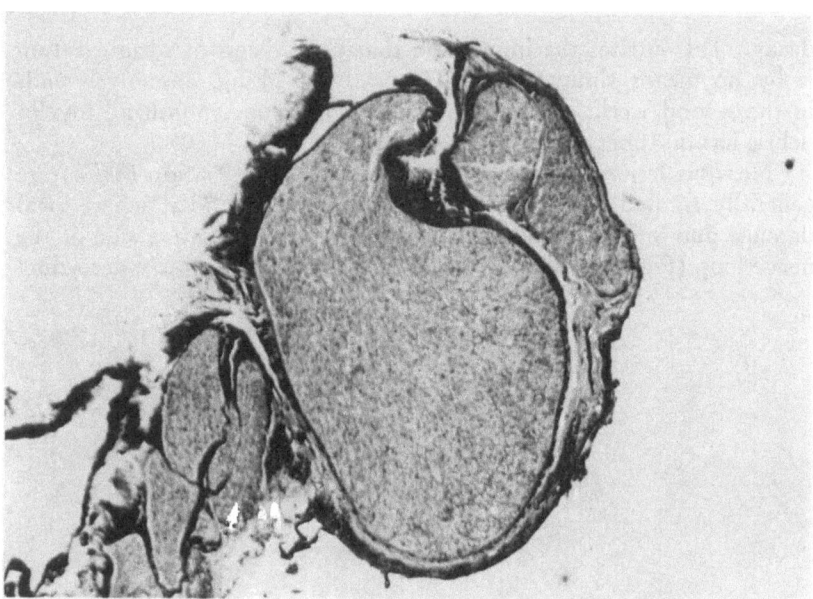

Fig. 19. Cross-section of a nerve hernia. Extensive haemorrhages in the ruptured outer integument. TG IV. 4th day. NS 2. Goldner. Magn. ×20.5

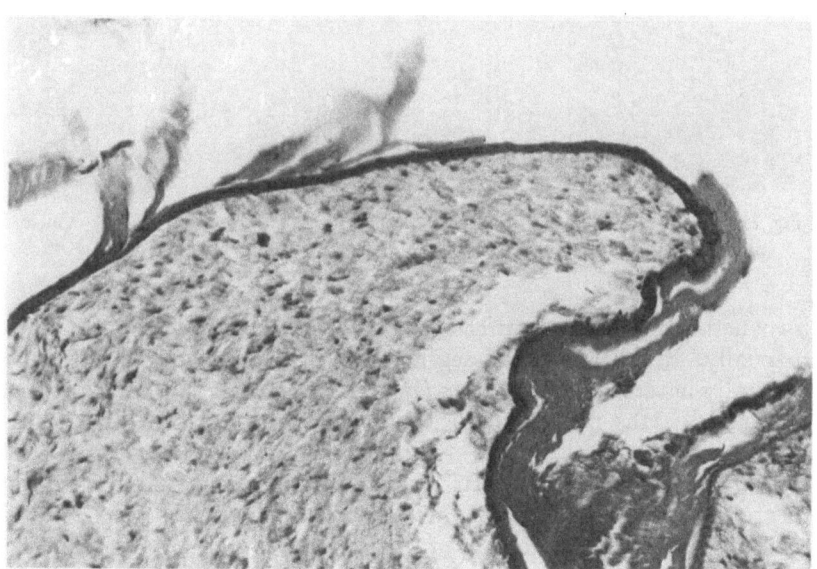

Fig. 20. Detail from Fig. 19. Rupture of the epineurium and of the adjacent superficial lamellae of the perineurium. Perineurial collagen layers still intact. TG IV. 4th day. NS 2. Van Gieson. Magn. ×51.2

3*

decay. This creates the impression that the process of disintegration is by no means simultaneous. Generally speaking, axonolysis ends in the second week, and by the end of the second month all myelin debris has disappeared.

Nervous lesions caused by the lowest degree of strain (TG I) are generally limited to the bottleneck around the cylinder, where local damage due to compression occurs mainly on the concave side of the nerve loop (Fig. 21). The extent of these injuries may vary according

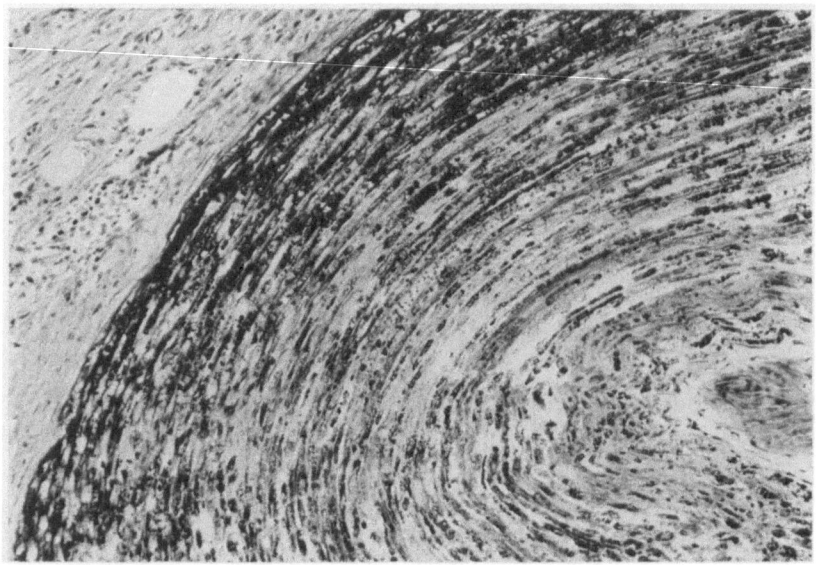

Fig. 21. Compression injury involving progressive demyelination of the concave side (right) of the nerve loop. TG I. 1st week. Klüver-Barrera. Magn. ×40

to whether the nerve is affected over its entire cross-section or only partially. In other cases the degeneration of the parenchyma extended centrally beyond the nerve loop (Fig. 22 b).

Initially, the process of degeneration under TG II–V is quickest and most intensive in the cylinder region and later progresses proximally and distally. Its centripetal extent is related to the degree of strain as well as to the individual elastic properties of each nerve (Fig. 23). The length of the injury to the proximal nerve segment increases with the degree of strain. It varies between individuals subjected to the same degree of strain. From strain group to strain group, the percentage of sciatic nerves suffering from extreme central injuries increases. Of all individuals subjected to the lowest degree of strain (TG I), the sciatic nerve was damaged in the cylinder segment in 92% of all cases and in 16% back to segment 1. In 8% of all cases there were no alterations at all (Fig. 22 a), whereas under the highest degree

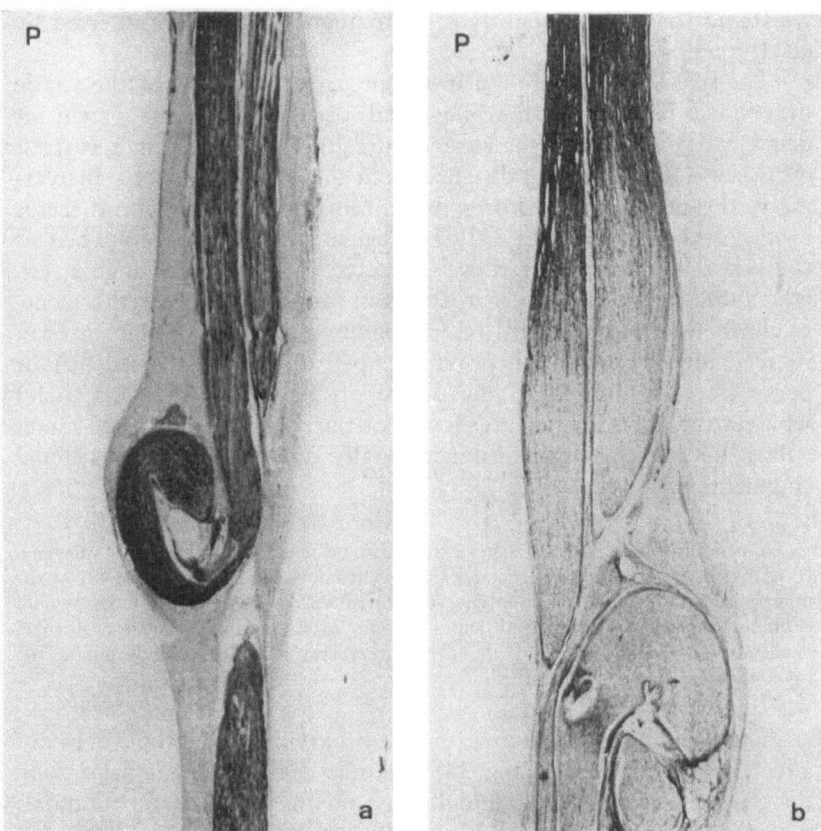

Fig. 22. Individual variation in the reaction of sciatic nerves to stretching by 2%. Cylinder region. a) No significant nerve change. TG I. 1st week. Klüver-Barrera. Magn. ×6.4. b) Extensive parenchymal degeneration over the entire nerve loop, ascending proximally. TG I. 1st week. Klüver-Barrera. P = proximally. Magn. ×10

of strain (TG V) segment 1 was injured in 100% of all cases, and segment 0, which is topographically on the level of the greater sciatic notch, was affected by stretch lesions in 63% of all cases (Table 4). The greater the extent of stretching, the lower became the number of nerves whose fibres were partially unaffected, even in the peripheral segments. Nerves of this kind were found in the following

proportions: TG I, 75%; TG II, 67%; TG III, 40%; TG IV, 29%;
TG V, 25%. Most of the nerve fibres remaining intact were isolated;
some survived in groups. The loss of intact nerve fibres causes a
marked rarefaction and dissociation of axons. The mechanical vulner-
ability of small diameter nerve fibres seems to be relatively low, for
we found that predominantly large diameter axons were affected by
all degrees of strain.

The stretch injuries found in the proximal segments of the sciatic
nerves exhibited some morphological peculiarities. The extent of
degenerative changes in the parenchyma gradually diminishes as stress
decreases with increasing distance from the cylinder region. Increasingly, the degeneration process is concentrated on the central sector
of the nerve, so that the field of degeneration can be described as
conical. The base of the cone is situated in the area of high stress,
where the entire nerve cross-section is affected. Above this zone,
a subperineurial ring of still-intact densely packed nerve filaments can
be recognized, and at the proximal apex of the cone the deficit of
nerve fibres is limited to the centre of the nerve (Fig. 24 a, b, c)
whereas the fibres in the outer layers of the nerve are preserved intact
over a longer centrifugal distance, finally dissolving into convoluted
fragments.

A proximal lesion of the same extent can be caused by secondary ischaemia.
It seems that the larger superficial vasa nervorum which are less affected by the
injury are still capable of supplying the surrounding parenchyma, which would
explain why the subperineurial axons remain intact over a longer centrifugal
distance. The central area of the nerve degenerates because circulation in the
inner nutrient vessels is disturbed.

The caudal traction acting on the proximal nerve trunk does not
affect its muscular rami (Fig. 25), the only evidence of damage being
the imperfect or missing undulation of the fibres as the branches
separate just before leaving the parent nerve (Fig. 26). Unlike the
main trunk, these branches are not affected by demyelination or
axonolysis, except for some individual nerve fibres close to the main
trunk which are affected by the stress because their sheaths are inter-
connected with those of the main trunk. Distally, the stress caused
by cranial traction affects the nerve branches as well. The shorter
these branches are compared to the main branches, i.e., the tibial and
peroneal nerves, the earlier and the more extensively they are affected
by the process of degeneration.

The subsequent regeneration of the parenchyma begins with a
dilatation of the proximal stumps of the axons. As distinct from
neurotomy, these growth bulbs will not appear until during the 4th

day and in comparatively much smaller numbers. Generally, they occur in nerve lesions of 2 and 4⁰/o elongation only. The proliferation of Schwann's cells, which precedes the terminal regeneration of axons, begins in the most intensely injured region. As the stretch injury

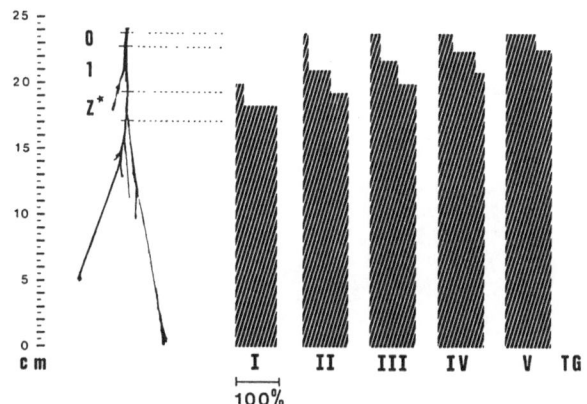

Fig. 23. Proximal and distal spread of nerve degeneration. Percentage of cases under various degrees of strain. Z* cylinder region (NS 2)

Table 4. *Spread of Lesions in the Proximal Nerve Segments Under Various Degrees of Strain. Percentage of Cases. Z* = cylinder region (NS 2)*

nerve segment

TG	Z*	1	0
I	92	16	0
II	100	59	9
III	100	60	20
IV	100	79	29
V	100	100	63

spreads proximally and distally, Schwann's cells also begin to move in the other affected segments. In some TG I cases, Schwann's cells began to proliferate after 4 days, but 1 week elapsed before proliferation in most cases. Sciatic nerves stretched by 4 to 10⁰/o (TG II–V) show a distinct formation of Schwann's cells after 2 weeks, although there is no regeneration of axons as yet. After a lapse of another

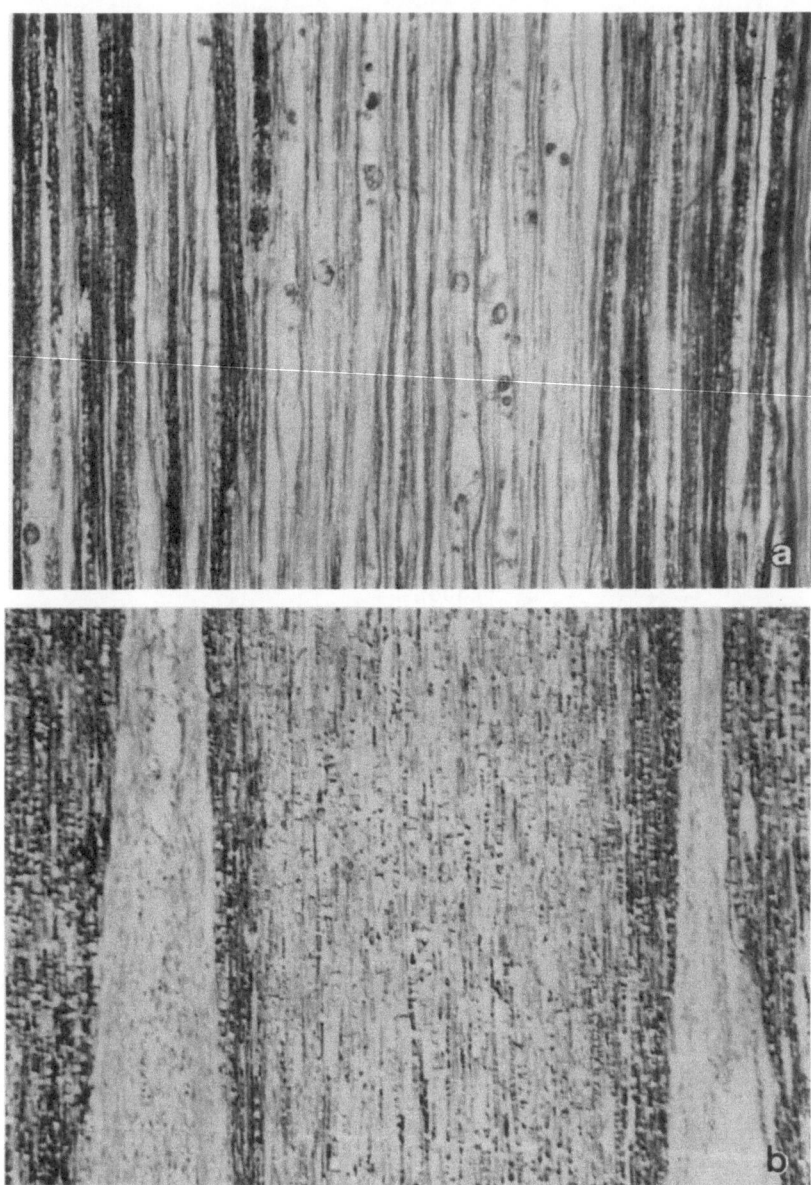

Fig. 24. Conical degeneration field in the proximal sciatic nerve trunk. a) Cone
apex showing partial loss of nerve fibres in the central zone of the nerve. TG IV.
13th week. NS 1. Klüver-Barrera. Magn. ×25.6. b) Central degeneration extending nearly to the outer fascicle layers. TG V. 4th day. NS 2. Klüver-Barrera.
Magn. ×25.6. c) Cross-section of the cone base. TG IV. 1st week. NS 0. Klüver-
Barrera. Magn. ×20.5

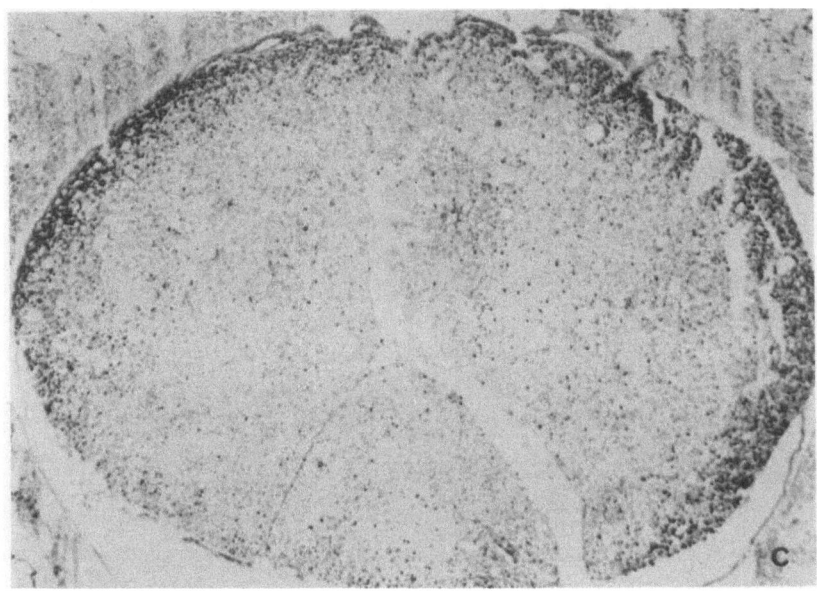

Fig. 24 c

week, the majority of TG III–V cases showed an activation of fibroblasts accompanied by collagenization (Fig. 27). Moderate endoneurial fibrosis occurred only in 1 out of all TG I and in 4 of the
TG II cases. It spread through the stressed nerve region, its density
varying regionally. The cross-sectional pattern of the nerve is not
extensively compromised by the axial proliferation of collagen fibres.
There is no undirected chaotic regeneration, as in cases of transitory
nerve elongation. Organization of extravasated blood only rarely
leads to a blockage of the nerve's longitudinal conduction. The endoneurial fibrosis recedes after the 13th week, but a sizeable amount of
collagen remains in the nerve even during the later stages of regeneration.

In our case, the regeneration of axons is delayed as compared to
neurotomy or the transitory stretching of nerves. The intervals elapsing before the sprouting of axon growth bulbs are prolonged in almost
direct proportion to the increase in strain. On an average, the process
of axon regeneration begins in TG I cases during the 2nd week, in
TG II cases during the 3rd week, and in TG III cases during the
4th week (Fig. 28). In some TG III cases it begins as early as the
2nd week. TG IV shows no evidence of new axons forming in the
4th week, but there is a similarity between these cases and TG V in

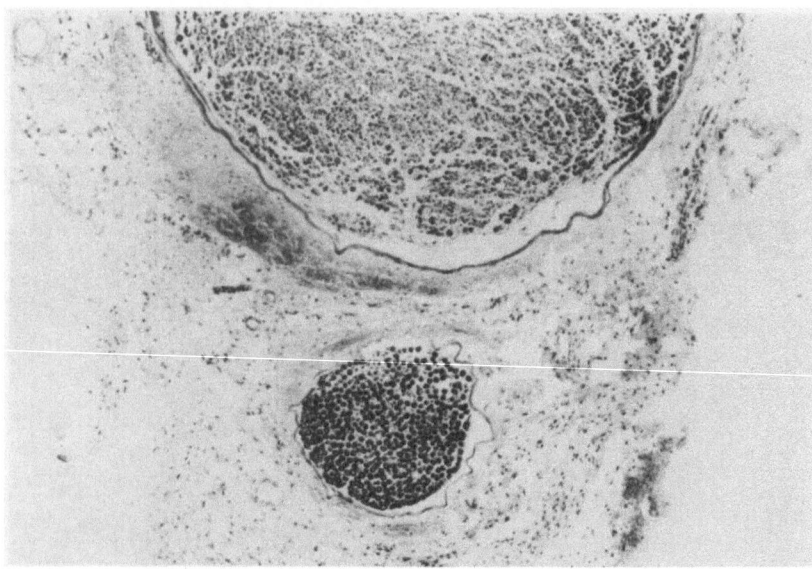

Fig. 25. Intact muscular ramus (bottom) and stretch-injured sciatic nerve trunk
(top). TG V. 8th week. NS 0. Klüver-Barrera. Magn. ×25.6

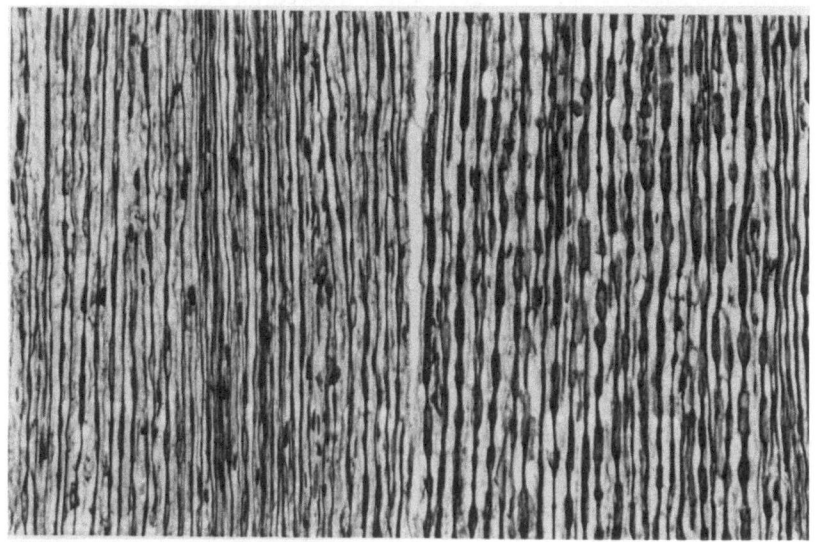

Fig. 26. Right: Normal configuration of axons in a branch already given off in
the sciatic nerve trunk. Left: Bundle of nerve fibres exposed to traction. TG IV.
13th week. NS 1. Bodian. Magn. ×64

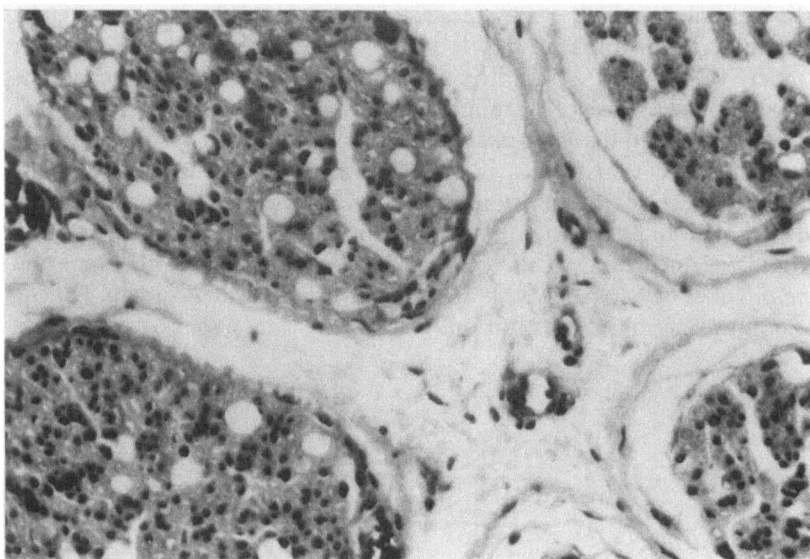

Fig. 27. Endoneurial fibrosis. Increase in the population of intrafascicular cells. Some of the larger Schwann's tubes are empty; most of them have shrunk and are constricted. TG III. 13th week. NS 4. Goldner. Magn. ×128

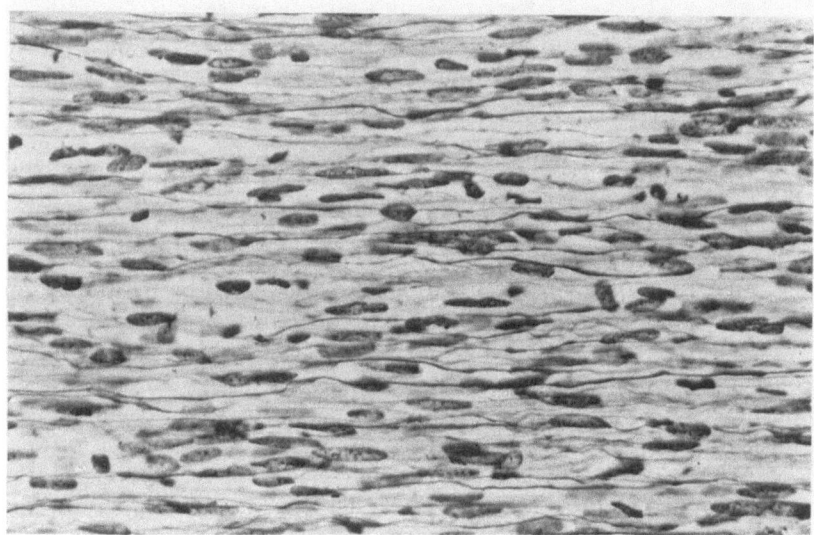

Fig. 28. Distal progression of axon regeneration. TG III. 8th week. NS 3. Bodian. Magn. ×128

that closely packed, regenerated thin axons reach segment 2 (the cylinder region) during the 8th week. We may therefore assume that under TG IV and V conditions axons begin to grow at some time during the 6th week. Terminally, the sprouting of axons begins at various sites in the proximal part of the nerve. This differs from neurotomy in that in this case the disruption of continuity and the origin of disintegration are not confined to one location only but are distributed over various levels, depending on the degree of strain applied. According to the configuration of the conical degeneration field, zones of neural growth are scattered more or less widely. During the initial periods of restitution, the regenerating axons in the central

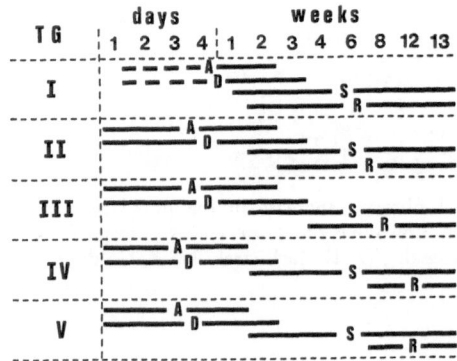

Fig. 29. Development of nerve degeneration related to the degree of chronic strain. *A* axonolysis; *D* demyelination; *S* proliferation of Schwann's cells; *R* regeneration of axons

and subperineurial areas are some distance apart proximally and distally, but this separation is eliminated as regeneration progresses. Fig. 29 shows the degeneration and regeneration history of chronically stretched sciatic nerves.

The speed of axon regeneration also proved to be dependent on strain, amounting in TG I and II to 3.28 mm/day, in TG III to 2.88 mm/day, and in TG IV and V to 1.42 mm/day. These figures only represent the rates of growth of the axon tips, without taking into account the latent period elapsed before the beginning of regeneration.

After a period of 1–2 weeks, the restitution of myelin sheaths follows the sprouting of axons. Under low degrees of strain, the first thin myelin mantles begin to appear during the 3rd and 4th week, whereas under the highest degree of strain (TG V) they appear during the 8th week. This indicates that there is also a relationship

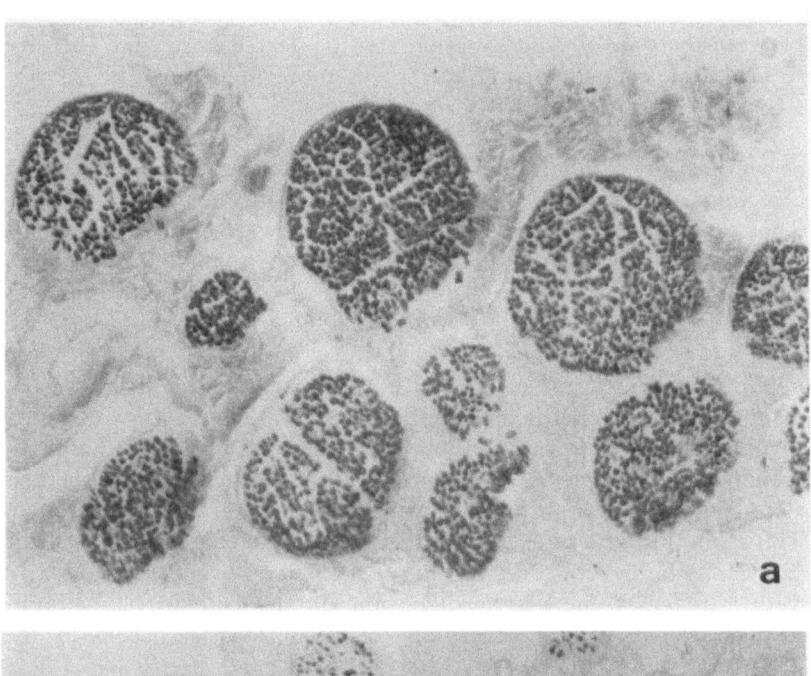

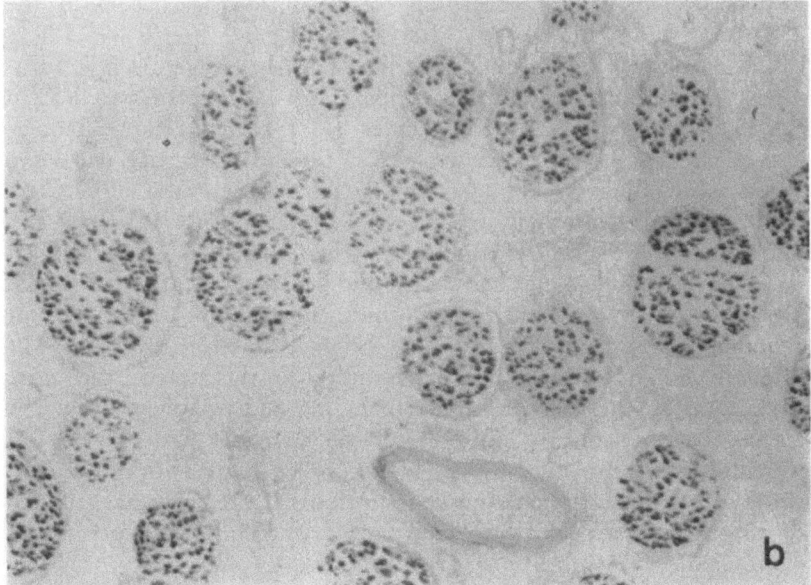

Fig. 30. Isomorphous pattern of regeneration with reduction of fascicle cross-sections. Remyelinated nerve fibres (b). TG II. 35th week. NS 4. Klüver-Barrera. Magn. ×40. Compare (a): Normal nerve cross-section on the same level and at the same magnification

between the time of remyelination and the degree of strain. The tube segments of young myelin sheaths are more numerous and shorter than those of normal nerve fibres.

Newly formed nerve fibres grow along Büngner's cellular bands as well as along longitudinally proliferated neural fibroblasts, their direction of growth being determined by intraneural stress lines. Thus, sprouting axons can bridge the gap between the retracted ends of ruptured endoneurial tubes, so that regeneration is isomorphous in spite of the discontinuity of the nerve fibres and sheaths which is produced by TG II–V (Fig. 30 a, b). Under TG I conditions, the presence of still-intact endoneurial tubes ensures that the original neural pattern is restored. The only justification for identifying TG I as an axonotmesis as defined by Seddon (1943) is the type of lesion involved. The endoneurial tubes are constricted because the cross-section of the nerve is mechanically reduced, and because there is some morphological shrinkage during degeneration and regeneration. This shrinking process is accompanied by a diameter reduction in the fascicles, which occurs even outside of high-stress zones (Fig. 30 b). In very rare cases there is a dilatation of the endoneurial sheaths, a phenomenon which, according to Piscol (1965), occurs in the peripheral stump immediately after neurotomy.

Despite continued chronic stretching and shrinkage of the integuments, the original undulation reappears in the neural as well as in the connective tissue elements. Under TG I–III conditions, undulation is restored by the 13th week over the entire regenerated nerve segment including the cylinder region. At this time, the nerve fibres newly formed in the loop around the cylinder do not yet show any undulation under TG IV conditions, whereas at TG V the zone of maximum stress does not show any undulation even after 30 weeks, although the axon calibre and the thickness of the myelin sheaths of a number of young nerve fibres has begun to increase by then. The original undulation, however, has returned by this time in the entire nerve outside the cylinder zone, including the periphery (Fig. 31). As the disappearance of fibre undulation coincides with the physiological elastic limit of a nerve (Nauck 1931), its reappearance in a chronically stretched sciatic nerve indicates that the nerve has adapted to continued stress and has overcome it by retaining a permanent elongation.

   b) Discussion: Nauck (1931), Schneider (1952), and Sunderland (1965) stated that one of the essential elements protecting the parenchyma from mechanical damage was the connective tissue sheath of a nerve. In isolated nerve fibres, this protective function is performed by the endoneurial fibril sheath, in the fascicles by the perineurium, and in the nerve trunk, by the epineurium. This is not corroborated by our experiments, for the parenchyma, when chronically stretched, is clearly more vulnerable than the sheaths.

Our findings concerning the tensile strength of the various nerve tissue components are in agreement with those reported by Liu, Benda, and Lewey (1948), and Sunderland (1972) in connection with

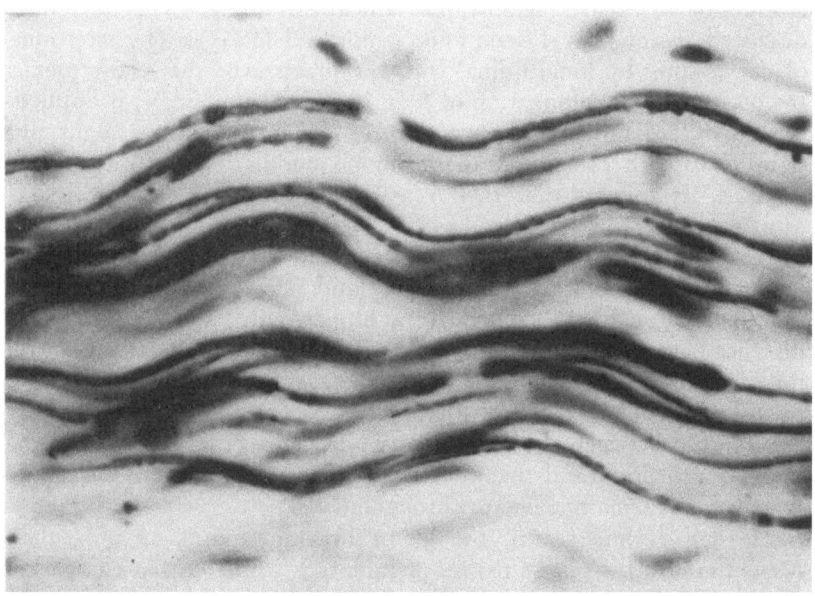

Fig. 31. Reconstitution of normal fibre undulation. Increase in myelin sheath thickness still minimal. TG V. 30th week. NS 5. Klüver-Barrera. Magn. ×160

human nerves excised from dead bodies, and with the results of the experiments performed by Schneider (1952) on isolated sciatic nerve fibres microsurgically excised from giant terrestrial frogs. During chronic stretching of the sciatic nerve, its epineurium often remains intact after a rupture of the perineurial sheath. However, the epineurium, being unable to protect the parenchyma when herniated because of the defect in the perineurium, cannot prevent lesional nerve degeneration.

Nerves can adapt to the usual direction of motion in the extremity, because, in a relaxed state, they are capable of providing extra length by having their anatomical course straightened (Sunderland 1965), by virtue of their fascicle undulations known as Nauck's striations (Schneider 1952, Sunderland 1965) and the undulations of

their individual fibres (Nauck 1931, Sunderland and Bradley 1961).
Nauck (1931) states that the physiological limit of elongation of a
nerve is reached as soon as its undulations are straightened out. In
the sciatic nerve of white mice, this limit is reached when the nerve
is elongated by 5 to 6%, and in the sciatic nerve of rabbits, this limit
corresponds to stretching by 2 to 4%. As early as 1943, Glees thought
that the Schmidt-Lantermann incisures of nerve fibres might serve as
a kind of safeguard against mechanical stretching. This idea was
discussed recently by Friede and Samorajski (1967). The stretching
of nerve fibres by longitudinal traction affects even the sciatic plexus
region if a chronic elongation of 8 or 10% (TG IV and V) is applied.
On the other hand, spinal nerve root fibres normally are straight and
parallel to each other and there are no undulations or plexus formations. It follows that their reaction to chronic stress is difficult
to assess.

Liu, Benda, and Lewey (1948), Hoen and Brackett (1956), Sunderland and Bradley (1961), and Sunderland (1972), in their studies of
stretched nerve fibres excised from human corpses, found that the
distance between the individual Ranvier's nodes had increased, which
indicated a lengthening of the internodal segments.

Schneider (1952) found that there is not necessarily a linear
relationship between the reduction of the nerve cross-section and the
increase in length, and that the width and the diameter of the nodal
fibre sections remain constant throughout.

Under chronic strain, the lower breaking point of individual
nerve fibres in the sciatic nerves of rabbits is reached at an elongation
of 4% (TG II). Similarly, in human nerves excised post mortem, the
breaking point, according to Liu, Benda, and Lewey (1948) is reached
at an elongation of 4.7%. In 1952, Schneider was able to establish
that stretched nerve fibres do not break where they are thinnest
(Ranvier's node) but always in their internodal segments. Schneider
(1952) thought that this high mechanical strength of the nodal region
of individual nerve fibres was due to the comparative thickness of the
fibril sheath in that location.

Multiple ruptures of nerve fibres in chronically stretched sciatic
nerves are due to the close connexion existing between the viscous
neurilemma and the elastic endoneurial sheath. The stretch behaviour
of the viscous components does not match that of the elastic structural components, so that the former will impede the entire process
and rupture at their interconnexions.

The fact that haemorrhages due to angiorrhexis are more frequent
in the outer nerve sheaths even after transitory stretching, starting
at an elongation of 6%, was confirmed by Takimoto (1916), and

Liu, Benda, and Lewey (1948). Similar to our own findings, Highet and Holmes (1943), Denny-Brown and Doherty (1945) found some vasa nervorum to display angiofibrosis, intimal proliferation, and thrombotic occlusions. Under chronic nerve strain, the spread of extravasated blood is limited, as the pressure inside the nerve increases continuously due to the reduction of its diameter. Local effects of these haemorrhages are mainly in the form of circulatory obstruction with ruptured blood vessels causing regional interruptions of the neural vascular network. In addition to direct mechanical injuries to the parenchyma, an increase in intraneural pressure causes compression of the vasa nervorum which, in turn, leads to diminished blood circulation and an impairment of the nutrient supply.

The intraneural pressure increase is impressively demonstrated by the herniation of the parenchyma. Once the connective tissue sheaths have ruptured, the only possible way of compensating for the continuously increasing pressure is towards the outside. Neural prolapses, just like those occurring after acute transitory traction of a nerve (Denny-Brown and Doherty 1945, Liu, Benda, and Lewey 1948, Sunderland 1972), are accompanied by a complete or partial rupture of the perineurium. According to Sunderland (1946), rupture of the perineurium alone will not cause herniation, the major factor determining the pathogenesis of the prolapse of the parenchyma and of the secondary Wallerian degeneration being the increase of intraneural pressure. The fact that the sciatic nerve trunk is evidently predisposed towards herniation can be explained by the fact that the tensile strength of any nerve increases with the number of its fascicles, i.e., with the proportional increase in perineurial and interfascicular connective tissue (Sunderland and Bradley 1952, Sunderland 1972). Chronic strain on the sciatic nerve of a rabbit will lead to rupture of the perineurium and herniation with an elongation of no more than 8% (TG IV), whereas transitory stretching led to herniation of the nerve from an elongation of 21% and upwards (Liu, Benda, and Lewey 1948), Denny-Brown and Doherty (1945) found herniation only after overextending the nerve by 100%.

Other permanently stretched nerves and their still-continuous perineurial sheaths are evidently also subjected to intraneural pressure whose increase depends on the momentary degree of strain. This seems to be corroborated by histological evidence obtained at elongations of TG II–V. X-ray contrast neurography provides an impressive demonstration of the high pressure level inside a stressed nerve (Fig. 32), which is due to the fact that the viscous tissue components located inside the nerve whose diameter is reduced by elongation are incompressible. Thus, all nerve fibres are subjected to direct compression and deformation. The extent of the compression effects develops parallel to the degree of strain and is evident over the entire nerve region which is under stress. As the strain increases, stress begins to make itself felt at increasing distances from the cylinder region, so that both the intensity and the proximal and distal spread of the compression injuries increase in proportion. The proximal and distal decrease of stress in a stretched nerve is due to static and sliding friction as well as to the fact that the nerve is fixed to the mesoneurium and to the effector organs by its branches.

In chronically stretched nerves, the process of parenchymal degeneration corresponds to the secondary Wallerian degeneration which occurs after neurotomy. However, not all nerve fibres will degenerate in every case. Those remaining unaffected are mostly of a thinner calibre. As early as 1903, Bethe stated: "It is mainly thin nerve fibres which most actively resist the process of degeneration." The fact that there are individual differences in the resistance of nerves to chronic straining even at the same degree of strain is documented by variations in the quantitative extent of fibre damage, in the number of intact axons, and in the proximal spread of the disintegration field. According to Sunderland and Bradley (1961) and Sunderland (1972), the lack of uniformity in the extensibility of nerves is caused by the following variables: Cross-sectional area, state of the tissue components, proportion of connective tissue, number of fascicles, structure of the inner plexus, and configuration of the vascular system.

Variations in the elastic properties of nerves as well as in the amount of strain to which they are subjected do not permit identical reduction of the cross-sectional area, so that the number of nerve fibres per unit area varies. This is one of the reasons why it is impossible to perform a quantitative analysis of, for instance, the relationship between the number of intact and the number of injured nerve fibres.

Simultaneous local compression injuries to the nerve in the cylinder strait are due to the reduction of the physiological range of extensibility which is caused even by elongations as low as 2⁰/₀ (TG I).

It is impossible for the nerves to be damaged by pressure from the adjacent muscular substance, as in this case the resultant changes in the nerve would have begun to appear in its outer convex regions. Compression caused by the weight of the cylinder itself could not possibly cause any damage either, as the implanted cylinder is fixed on both sides to the adjacent tissue, and its weight (0.195 g) is irrelevant. The probability of axial compression lesions is eliminated by the absence of a neutral, undamaged section of the parenchyma which would have to be located between the inner (concave) and the outer (convex) layers of the nerve loop. Any compression injuries in the cylinder region are due to the limited range of physiological extensibility; this is confirmed by the initial thinning of the connective tissue sheath on the convex side of the nerve as soon as the nerve is being moderately stretched. Although no stretching of the nerve is observed in the cylinder loop during the implantation of a cylinder 2 mm in diameter with the hip and knee joints flexed on an average by 90°, any extension of the extremity will immediately cause a noticeable stretching of the sciatic nerve, which is then pressed to the cylinder.

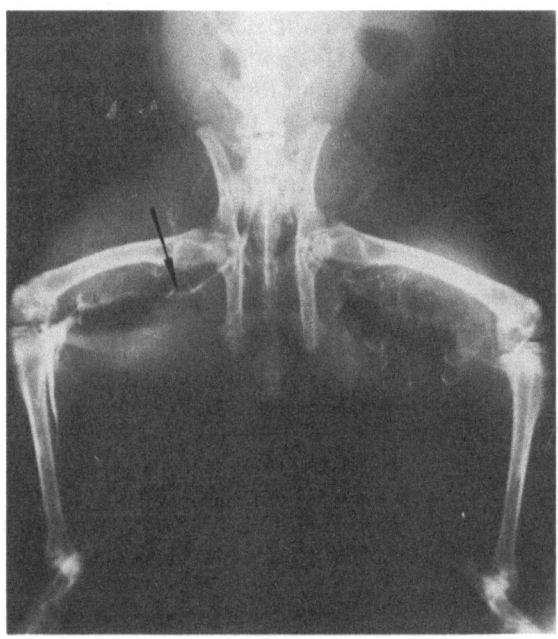

Fig. 32. Bilateral X-ray neurography of the sciatic nerve. Right extremity: Contrast medium in a normal nerve. Left extremity: Stretched nerve not perfused with contrast because of the high level of intraneural pressure (TG III)

The presence of stretching effects is demonstrated by the fact that 16% of all cases showed a retrograde spreading of parenchymal degeneration which extended much further than after neurotomy.

At TG I and TG II, the field of degeneration develops unilaterally because there is a difference between the mechanical stresses acting on each side. The outer bands of nerve fibres are subjected to a comparatively high tensile load, whereas the inner ones which are in contact with the cylinder are subjected to a load just within the limit of tolerance.

Under TG III–V, the proximal trunk of the sciatic nerve shows a few isolated nerve fibres surviving intact in the cone-shaped field of degeneration, in addition to those surviving in the subperineurial region. It seems that a nutrient supply sufficient to cover the metabolic demand of these fibres is ensured by transfer of substances from the interstitial liquid, by increased permeability especially of the superficial vascular plexus (Olsson 1966, Mellick and Cavanach 1967, 1968), and because of the instability of the perineurial diffusion barrier, even if local circulation has come to a standstill.

Under TG I and TG II, terminal axon bulbs indicating regeneration do not begin to appear until the fourth day and are nearly completely absent under TG III–V, whereas, according to Kreutzberg (1971), the latent period after neurotomy does not exceed 3 to 4 days. In our case, this phenomenon is due to the high intraneural pressure which impedes the continued supply of axoplasm to the nerve fibres. Depending on the degree of strain, the interval elapsing before the sprouting of naked axons is 2–8 weeks, whereas it amounts to 3–7 days in a severed nerve (Gutmann 1958, Wechsler and Hager 1962, Hanefeld 1966, Hager 1968, Kreutzberg 1971). The speed of axon growth amounts to 3.28 mm/day under lesser and to 1.42 mm/day under greater chronic strain, which indicates a distinct reduction of growth compared to the rates obtained after distal and proximal neurotomy of the sciatic nerve (4.11 ± 0.4 mm/day and 4.48 ± 0.3 mm/day). Axon regeneration is impeded to an extent depending on the prevalent stress, and axons can only sprout freely after the nerve has nearly adapted to this. Another factor impeding axonal regeneration is the ischaemia which is caused by the strain. Both Weddell (1942) and Causey (1955) found that nerve fibres located close to unaffected blood vessels will regenerate fastest.

Remyelination under chronic strain commences 1–2 weeks after the sprouting of axons (TG I: 3rd–4th week, TG V: 9th week). Takimoto (1916) observed a regeneration of myelin as early as 2 weeks after transitory traction applied to the sciatic nerve, whereas Rexed and Swensson (1940) and Young (1942) reported it during the third week after neurotomy.

The intrafascicular proliferation of mesenchymal tissue can be said to be a reaction to continuous tensile loading. It is a mechanically compensatory process which stabilizes the nerve. Highet and Sanders (1943) regard the presence of fibroblastic proliferation and of collagen formation as an important histological finding in the differentiation between stretched and non-stretched nerves. Moreover, the increase of Schwann's cells seems to be greater in a stretched nerve than in the proximal stump of a nerve sutured end-to-end free of tension (Highet and Sanders 1943). Among the aetiological factors causing the production of collagen in a nerve are: ischaemia, stress, lack of parenchymal regeneration, and aging (Denny-Brown and Doherty

1945). Experiments made under chronic strain confirm that the extent of connective tissue proliferation depends on the degree of strain applied.

In a stretched nerve, the endoneurial fibroblasts will migrate in a proximal and distal direction along the lines of stress (Highet and Holmes 1943, Highet and Sanders 1943), thus establishing the prerequisite for the longitudinal conduction of sprouting axons. The presence of a constant tensile load and of parallel axial lines of tension as well as the high level of intraneural pressure make it well-nigh impossible for the intrafascicular tissue including the recovering parenchyma to move transversely, so that there can be no noticeable change in the pattern of distribution. A different situation prevails after stretch injuries involving total rupture of the outer sheaths and herniation of their contents. However, there is no development of pseudoneuromas.

Holmes and Young (1942) as well as Sanders and Young (1944) indicated that shrinkage of endoneurial tubes might impede the regeneration of nerve fibres. On the other hand, the experiments made by Sunderland and Bradley (1950) prove that the distal stump of a severed nerve retains for at least 12 months the capacity of regenerating by allowing new nerve fibres to grow.

The fact that regenerated nerve fibres will regain their original undulation even under a permanent longitudinal strain of 10% (TG V) proves that peripheral nerves can adapt to constant tensile loading extremely well and that the state of stress in the nerve has disappeared. The period of time required for this process varies largely with the degree of strain applied. Moreover, the reappearance of undulation demonstrates that chronically stretched nerves do not develop plastic properties after the repair of the lesion but renew their capacity for elongation and thus their elastic quality.

2. Vasa Nervorum

a) Findings: The functional quality of peripheral nerves depends on the connexion between nerve fibres and parent ganglion cell bodies as well as on a continued and sufficient nutrient supply through the blood vessels.

Chronic stretching of a nerve produces ischaemia, the proximal and distal spread of which is proportional to the degree of strain applied. Depending on their intensity, stress and intraneural pressure either block or reduce the perfusion of the vascular system of the injured nerve segment with staining agents. By measuring, we found the lengths of ischaemic sections given in Table 5. Ischaemia always spreads symmetrically from the point of application of the tractive force. There is no difference between the peroneal and the tibial division, and there is no relationship to the segmental vascularisation of the sciatic nerve. Under TG II, ischaemia extends centripetally beyond the theoretical resection length, reaching to where the branches to the thigh muscles leave the parent nerve under TG III. Its extent increases with the degree of strain. As traction acts distally on the proximal sciatic nerve, only the trunk is stretched, whereas its muscular ramifications are compressed axially, so that their vasa nervorum can still be demonstrated by perfusion with Skriptol.

Figs. 33 a, b and 34 a, b show comparisons between a stretched and an unstretched nerve taken from the same animal. In the

Table 5. *Length of Ischaemic Nerve Segment Expressed in Absolute Figures and as a Percentage. Relation to Physical Data at Various Degrees of Strain (I = ischaemic nerve segment; L = total length of the sciatic nerve; TG = degree of strain; U = circumference of the cylinder; ε = strain; σ = stress)*

L [mm]	TG	U [mm]	ε [%]	σ $\frac{k\,p}{m\,m^2}$	I [m m]	I [%]
319,0 ± 11,9	I	6,28	1,97	0,028	0–10	0–3,1
	II	12,57	3,94	0,056	2 5	7,8
	III	18,85	5,91	0,083	40–55	12,5–17,2
	IV	25,13	7,88	0,111	60–70	18,8–21,9
	V	31,42	9,85	0,139	8 0	25,1

stretched nerve, the deep as well as the superficial vascular systems are deformed. Vessels are stretched and rarefied, and their lumina have been reduced in proportion to the degree of strain applied.

There are hardly any observations concerning either vessels entering obliquely or intraneural transverse anastomoses.

It is always the deep arterial network which is disturbed first, the superficial perineurial and epineurial blood vessels being affected later as the strain increases. Unimpaired deep blood vessels are never found when there is a defective superficial vascular plexus. Under TG IV and V, circulation is interrupted throughout the entire vascular system (Fig. 35 a), namely in all areas of high stress.

As stress decreases proximally and distally, the vascular system of the stretched nerve begins to operate again from level to level, starting in the superficial zones and ending with the central part of the nerve. As soon as stress is reduced to a certain low level, the vascularity of the nerve becomes normal (Fig. 35 b). In one TG I case, the vasculature was not compromised at all.

b) Discussion: Histopathological evidence concerning the parenchyma matches the various ischaemic states of stretched nerves. One finds degenerations directly caused by mechanical failure and lesions indirectly caused by ischaemia. However, it was impossible

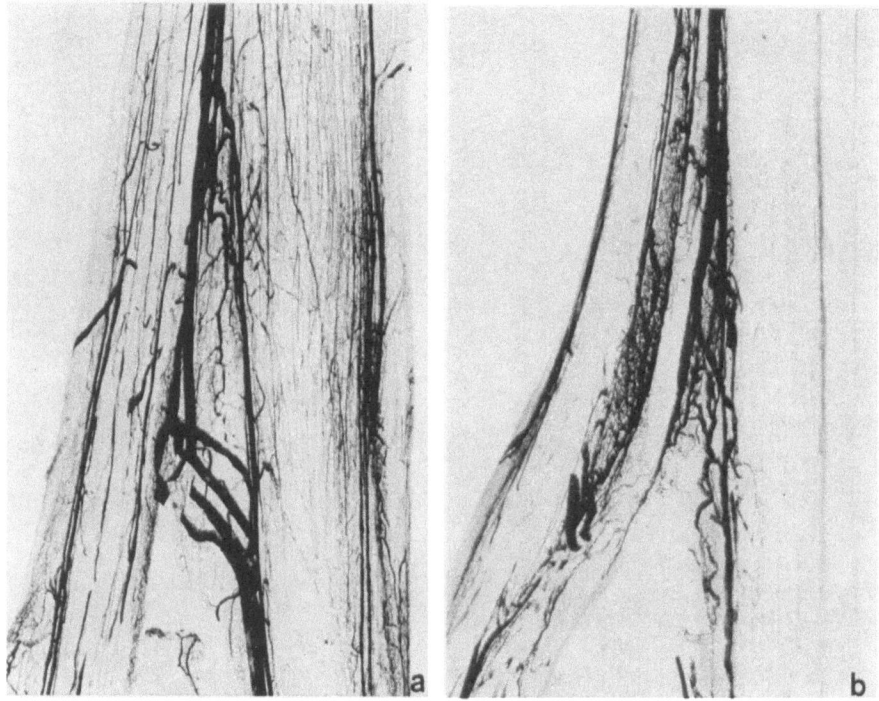

Fig. 33. Configuration of blood vessels in the sciatic nerve trunk and muscular branch. NS 1. Perfusion with Skriptol. Magn. ×5. a) Normal; b) TG IV. 1st day

to determine with sufficient clarity the extent of their influence on variations in the intensity of nerve lesions caused by the same stress. Stresses as low as 0.028 to 0.056 kp/mm² will compromise the blood circulation of the sciatic nerve. Stretched nerves are affected by disturbances of circulation resulting from a reduction in the lumina of the vasa nervorum caused by stretching, as well as by disturbances caused by compression of the blood vessels. Sunderland (1972), Lundborg and Rydevik (1973) already mentioned vascular compression due to high intraneural pressure. Interruption of transverse anastomoses is caused by shearing due to the unequal extensibility of the various tissues composing a nerve.

Numerous experimental studies and clinical observations have established the detrimental influence of ischaemia on the function and morphology of peripheral nerves. Our findings removed any doubt that vascular lesions provide an additional factor in producing injuries to the parenchyma of a permanently stretched nerve.

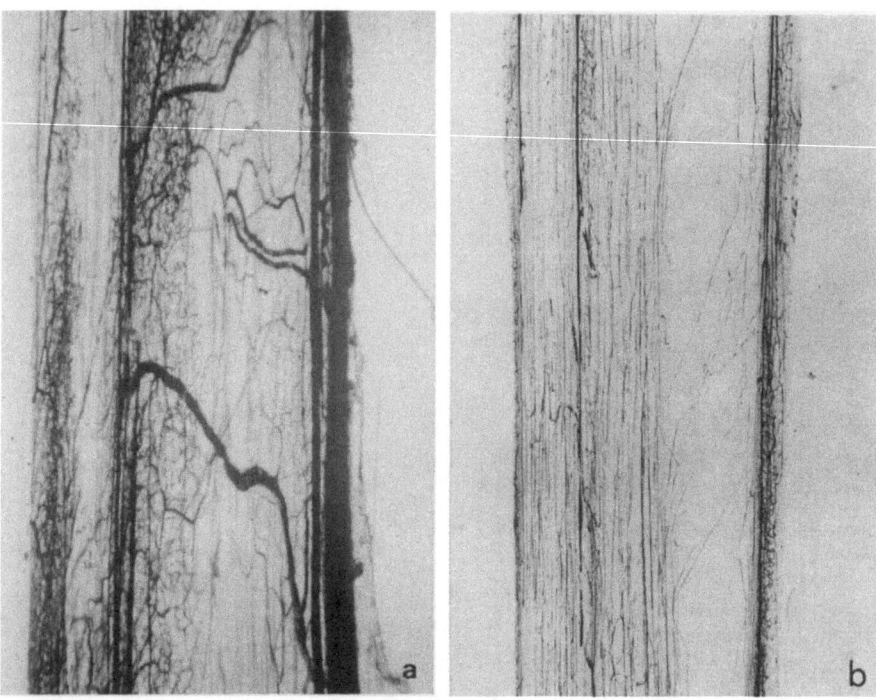

Fig. 34. Vascular system of the proximal sciatic nerve 15 mm below the muscular branch. NS 1. Perfusion with Skriptol. Magn. ×5. a) Normal; b) TG III. 1st day

3. Nerve Root

a) Findings: As traction acts peripherally on the proximal segment of the sciatic nerve it is likely that, depending on the strain, the sciatic plexus and the corresponding nerve and spinal roots will be mechanically affected as well. This influence may be enhanced by dynamic loading of the sciatic nerve caused by movements of the extremity.

Permanent stretching of the sciatic nerve causes mechanical traction which leads to injuries to the L 7 and S 1 nerve roots where they pass through the intervertebral foramina. These lesions are: Club-shaped swellings of the axons (Fig. 36), segmental demyelination

(Fig. 37), and endoneurial fibrosis of varying extent (Fig. 38). They begin to occur under TG II, and their incidence increases with the degree of strain. Under TG V, axon swellings and segmental disintegration of the myelin sheaths will appear as early as the 4th day (around the 7th day at lesser degrees of strain), whereas endoneurial fibrosis appears around the 8th week.

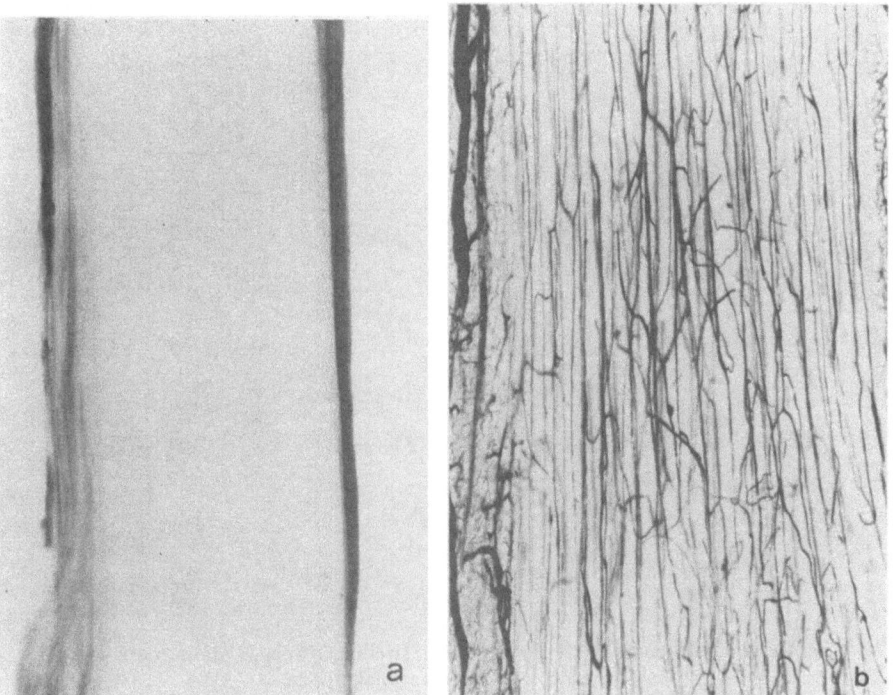

Fig. 35. a) No identification of the vasa nervorum. Tissue of the outer sheath merely diffusely tinged with Skriptol. TG IV. 1st day. NS 2. Magn. ×12.8. b) Regular intraneural vascular system. TG I. 1st day. NS 1. Perfusion with Skriptol. Magn. ×12.8

Segmental demyelination and beaded axons always appear simultaneously in the same circumscribed portion of a nerve. Continuity of the fibres is preserved; there are no newly sprouted axons. Interstitial root oedema may occur occasionally, most of it during the initial application of high degrees of strain.

In spite of the theoretical possibility of the stress spreading via the lumbosacral plexus, adjacent nerve roots not belonging to the sciatic nerve are not affected mechanically.

b) Discussion: Axon swellings and segmental demyelination, which we found at the nerve roots, have also been observed close to fresh as well as older lesions to central nerve fibres caused by mechanical factors (Bielschowsky 1906, Schlote 1961, Kreutzberg 1963) as well as by so-called degenerative diseases (Cajal 1904, Eicke 1957, Jakob 1957, Seitelberger 1957, Seitelberger and Gross 1957, Wohlfahrt 1959, Schlote 1961, Hager 1966). Distinct swellings were also observed in axons whose continuity had been preserved intact

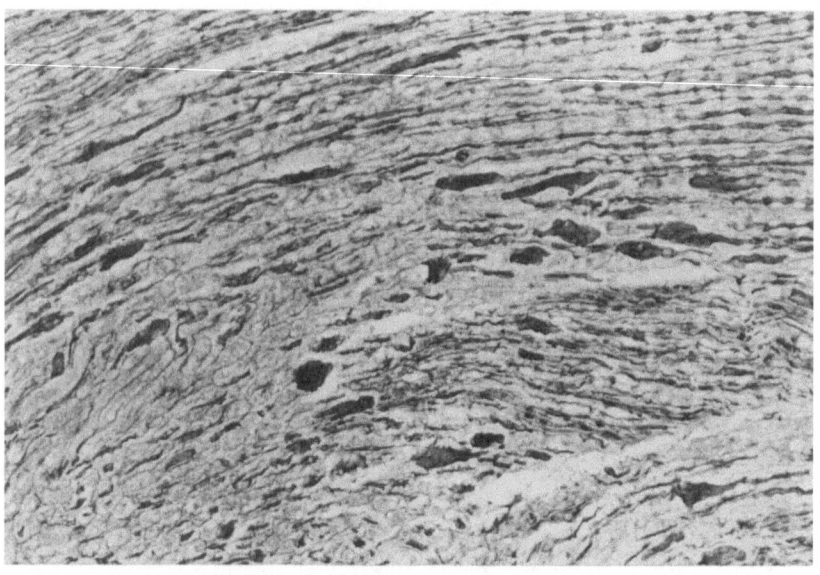

Fig. 36. Plaque and spindle-shaped axon swellings. Spinal nerve root. TG III.
8th week. Bodian. Magn. ×52

in the wound margin of severed long fibres of the spinal cord (Kreutzberg 1963). There may be a connection between these swellings and the patho-physiological processes involved in the repair of a wound (Kreutzberg 1963, cf. Heller, Wolfe, and Hesse 1962). Similar axon formations were described by Bielschowsky (1906) as occurring in areas of compression in the spinal cord, and by Schlote (1961) occurring in the margin of traumatic tissue injuries to the human brain.

It is probable that these nerve elongation findings are also influenced by mechanical factors. The morphological changes in the spinal roots are obviously due to compression as well as to impaired mobility, because a stretched nerve passes through its intervertebral

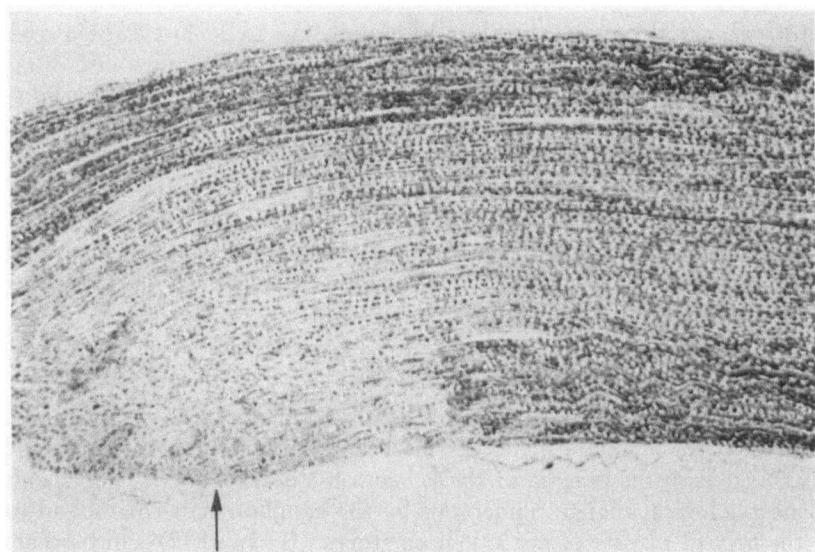

Fig. 37. Circumscribed site of segmental demyelination. Spinal nerve root. TG III. 8th week. Klüver-Barrera. Magn. ×16

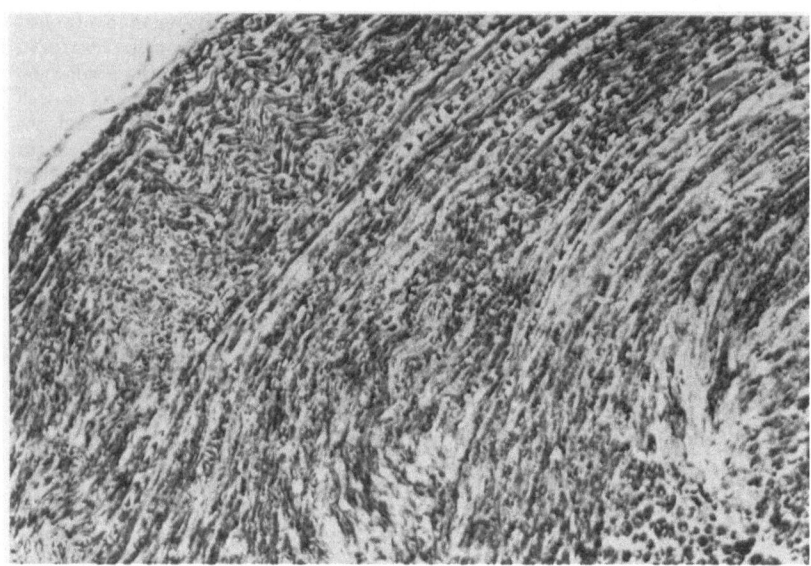

Fig. 38. Focal endoneurial collagenization. Spinal nerve root. TG III. 8th week. Goldner. Magn. ×40

foramen as through a bottleneck. According to Denny-Brown and Doherty (1945), neural oedema associated with transitory stretching of a nerve is caused by damage to small blood vessels in the endoneurium accompanied by tissue transudation. This causes fibroblastic proliferation within the oedematous nerve (Denny-Brown and Doherty 1945). As chronic stretching of the sciatic nerve produces much less root oedema than endoneurial fibrosis, the proliferation of connective tissue must be due to another cause, which we consider to be the fact that the nerve root is affected mechanically where it passes through the intervertebral foramen.

4. Spinal Cord and Spinal Ganglia

a) Findings: All degrees of strain applied to the sciatic nerve affected the parent cell bodies in the anterior columns of the spine as well as in the ganglia of the L 7 and S 1 dorsal roots. The various morphological changes undergone by the ganglion cells correspond to the typical picture of central chromatolysis (Nissl 1892) which occurs mainly after severance of axons (Heidenhain 1911, Spatz 1921, Scholz 1957, Krücke 1974, *et al.*) and which is sometimes followed by cellular atrophy.

The first reactive phenomena observed in neurones are perikaryon swelling and chromatolysis. The nucleus shifts to the periphery of the cell (Fig. 39). Recovery and restitution of the original cell picture are marked by reaggregation of Nissl substance and by a return of the nucleus to the centre of the cell. However, any overtaxing of the capacity for compensation of the nucleus and the perikaryon may result in cytolysis (Fig. 40 a, b), which is found in the spinal ganglia as well as in the anterior horns (Fig. 41). The intensity of this development and the extent of cellular changes are to some degree dependent on strain and on the proximal and distal spread of the nerve stretch injury, which varies in individual cases. Not all nerve fibres affected by a lesion will cause the parent cell bodies to react, so that individual cells may prove to be completely intact. The eventual tendency towards either cellular decay or restitution seems to be dependent on the distance between the cell body of an axon and the site of its injury.

Retrograde cellular reactions become evident around the 4th day, reaching their peak in the spinal ganglia after 1 week and in the anterior horns during the 4th to the 6th week. During the initial stage (4th–8th day), for instance, the quantitative proportion of nerve cells with their nuclei off centre is 1 : 3 between TG I and TG V, and 1 : 1.8 between TG I and TG IV. We arrived at these figures by counting 25 analogous section preparations per animal for each degree of strain applied. Restitution starts during the third week. Regressive changes start in the spinal ganglion cells around the 4th week, and in the anterior horn cells around the 8th week.

b) Discussion: It is only very rarely that histological analyses of indirect secondary changes in the anterior horn cells and in the spinal ganglia were made in connection with a stretched nerve (Takimoto

1916, Hoen and Brackett 1956). The findings of these analyses in no way contradicted the norm. The only mention made in the literature of the possibility of sciatic nerve cell bodies showing a retrograde reaction to nerve stretching occurs in the work of Takimoto (1916), who quotes Tarnomsky as stating that he had found the motor cells of the anterior horn chromatolytic and reduced in number.

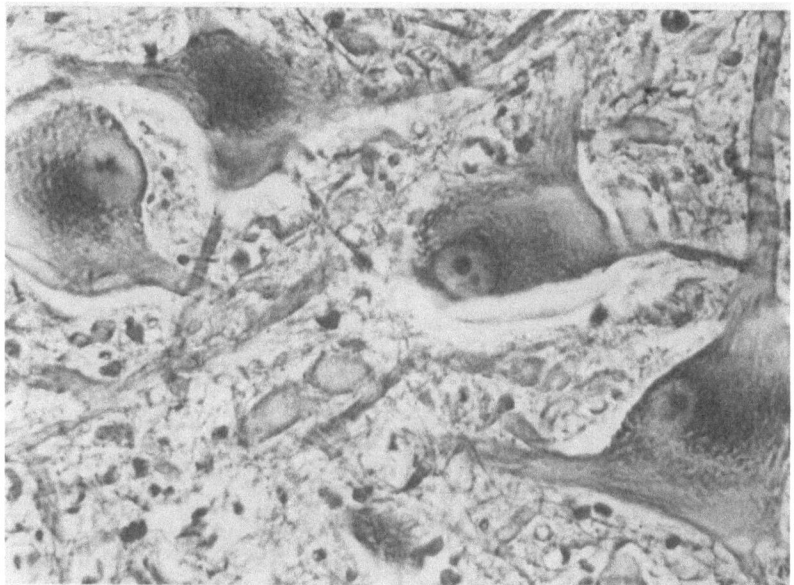

Fig. 39. Nuclei displaced towards the periphery of the cell. Anterior column. S 1. TG II. 2nd week. Bodian. Magn. ×160

As chronically stretched nerves are affected by a conical field of degeneration, which means that injured nerve fibres occur proximally at various levels, the restitution requirements vary from one cell to another. This explains why not all original cells react, and why they do not react uniformly. However, there is no quantitative uniformity even after neurotomy, because not all severed nerve fibres necessarily lead to a change in the parent cell body.

5. Muscles

a) Findings: During the early stage of permanent stretching of the sciatic nerve, uniform atrophy and a relative increase in the number of nuclei are observed throughout the entire muscle cross-section at all degrees of strain. These

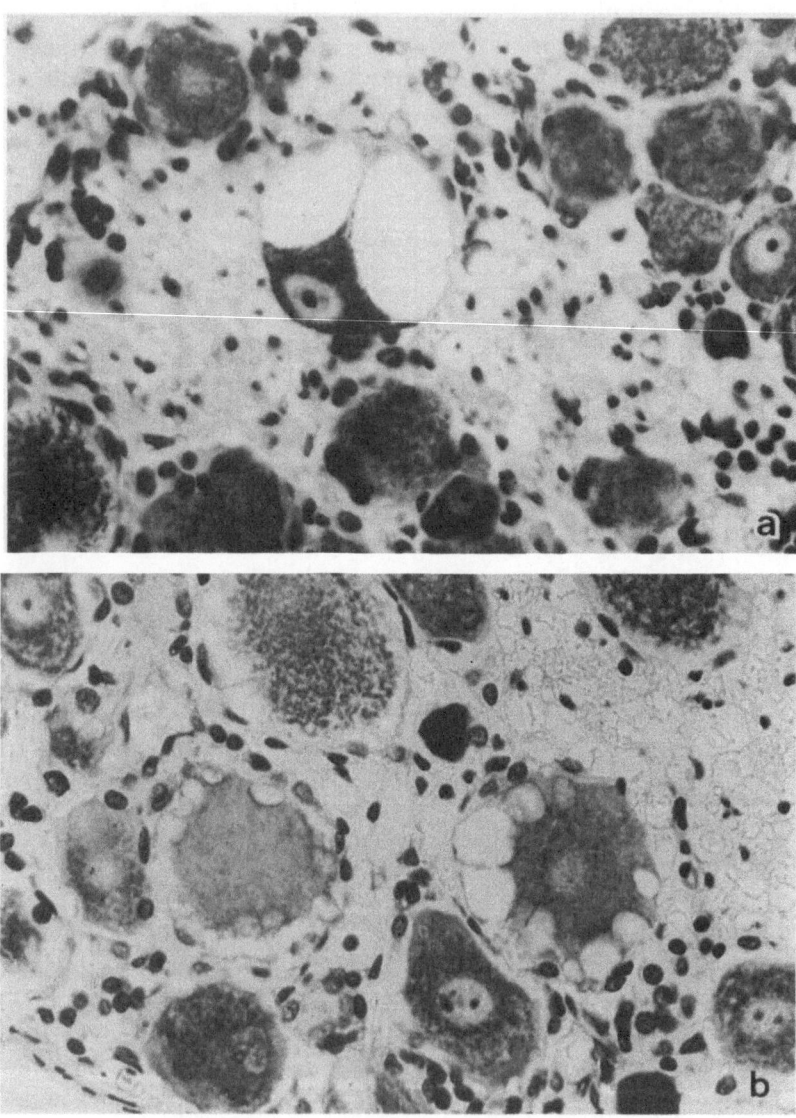

Fig. 40. Vacuolar degeneration of nerve cells. a) Anterior column. S 1. TG IV.
8th week. Nissl. Magn. ×160. b) Spinal ganglion. L 7. TG IV. 8th week. Nissl.
Magn. ×160

same phenomena even occurred in animals which were not affected by paresis and analgesia either initially or later. Later on, the originally polygonal fibres are found to have been replaced by rounded and largely hypertrophied fibres distributed in groups. These changes begin during the 2nd week under TG I and II, around the 3rd and 4th week under TG III, and around the 4th to 8th week under TG IV and V.

The appearance of hypertrophic muscle fibres is accompanied by a developing group atrophy (Fig. 42). However, uniform muscle atrophy continues in some cases (Fig. 43). The ratio between the quantity of atrophied and of hypertrophied fibres found in a muscle cross-section is not always dependent on the degree of

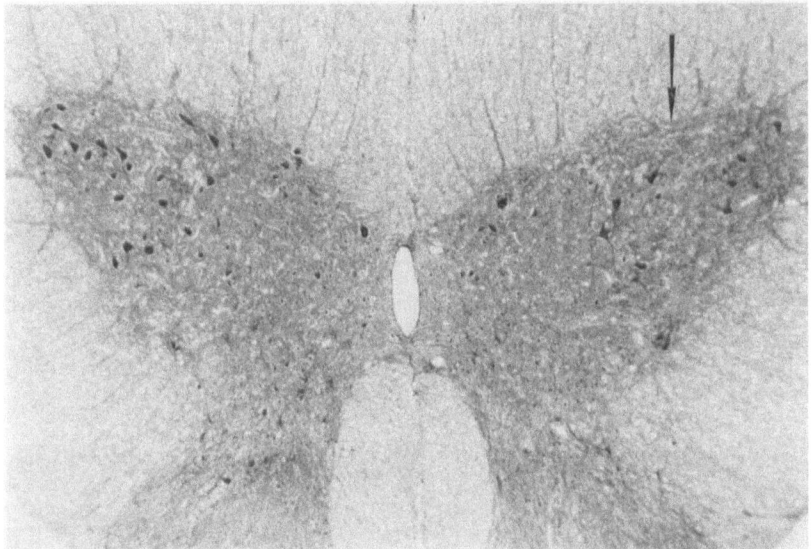

Fig. 41. Retrograde loss of cells in the left anterior horn (right). TG II. 35th week. Bodian. Magn. ×10

strain. Ratios will fluctuate even within one degree of strain. Generally speaking, atrophied muscle fibres are more numerous during the later stages of TG III–V.

Hypertrophied muscle fibres show the following myopathic changes: An increase in the number of centrally located nuclei (up to 14), and vacuolation. In addition to vacuolar degeneration, some instances of hyalinosis and central fibre necrosis were observed (Fig. 44 a, b, c).

In addition to these secondary changes, interstitial fibrosis was increasingly found during the 4th to 6th week. Atrophy, which hitherto had been generalized and uniform, began to show considerable indications of scleromatosis during the 8th week. This may either lead to pseudo-lobulation (Fig. 45), or else the process may turn cirrhotic. Some instances of lipomatous transformation were found during the later stages.

From the 13th week onwards, the affected muscular tissue was found to contain spindle-shaped myoblasts, which fused and grew into muscle tubes running parallel to the original direction of the fibres. These tubes, which indicate regeneration, will occur even in denervated muscle tissue and under high degrees of strain.

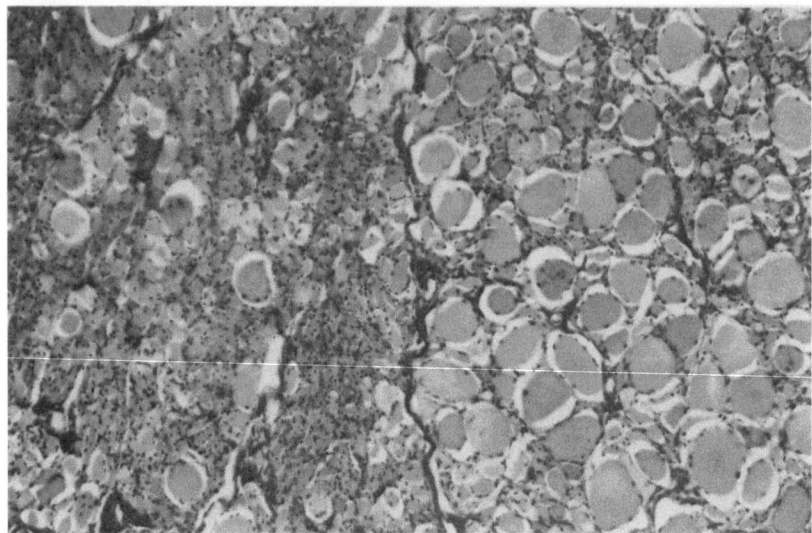

Fig. 42. Fields of muscular denervation atrophy showing some sites of marked hypertrophy of the fibres of the remaining parenchyma. TG III. 13th week. Van Gieson. Magn. ×40

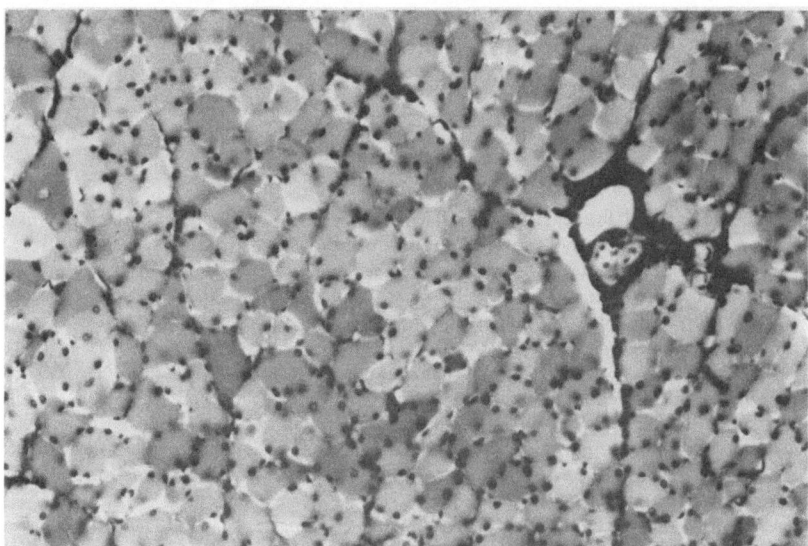

Fig. 43. Simple generalized muscular atrophy involving a relative increase in the number of sarcolemmal nuclei. TG I. 4th week. Van Gieson. Magn. ×82

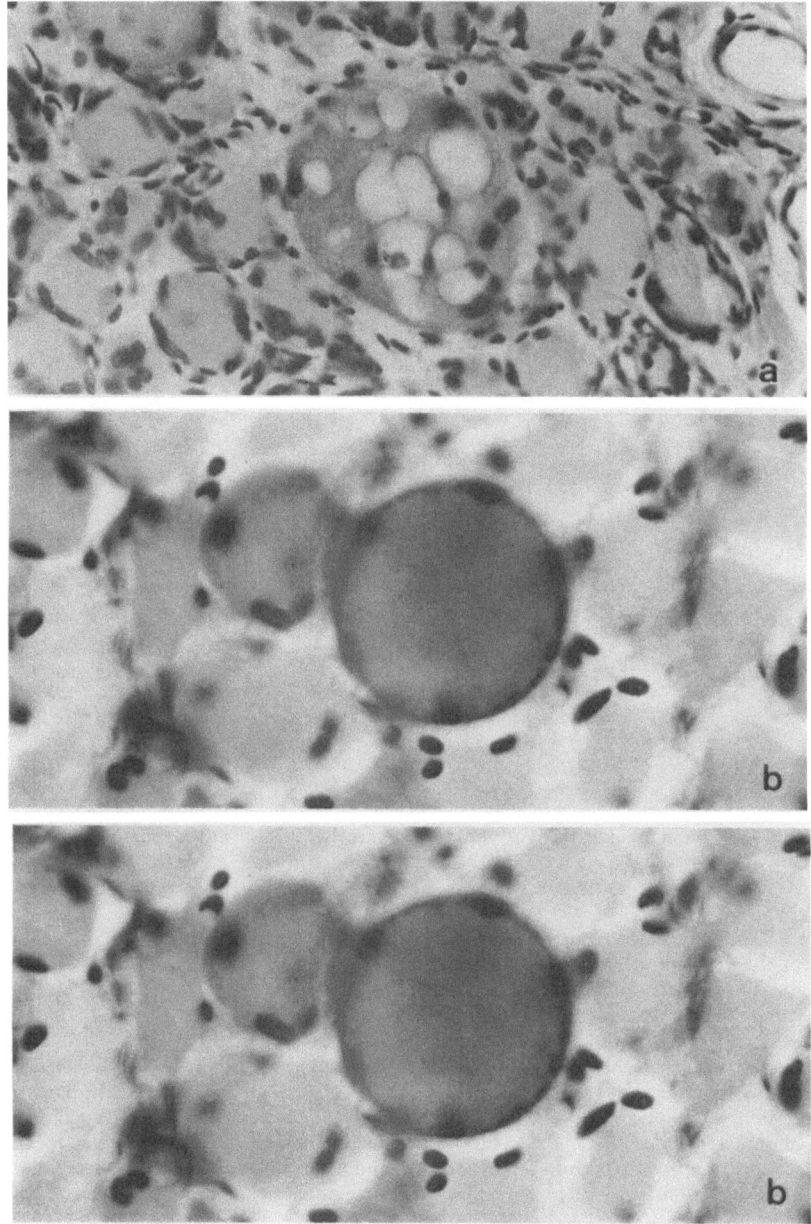

Fig. 44. Myopathic changes. a) Vacuolar degeneration. TG IV. 13th week. Van Gieson. Magn. ×128. b) Hyaline degeneration. TG I. 6th week. Van Gieson. Magn. ×256. c) Central fibre necrosis. TG I. 4th week. Van Gieson. Magn. ×256

b) Discussion: Whenever a case of histologically uniform atrophy occurred in one of our experiments, it was a disuse atrophy brought about by the inactivity of the extremity after operation extending beyond the normal period of traumatic and stretching pain. This prolongation was caused by a persistent feeling of discomfort brought about by the implantation of a foreign body, *i.e.*, the cylinder. It is impossible to differentiate between a disuse atrophy and a denervation atrophy due to extensive stretch injuries to the nerve. The electron microscopy findings of Wechsler and Hager (1960, 1961, 1962) showed experimentally that disuse and denervation atrophy are absolutely identical.

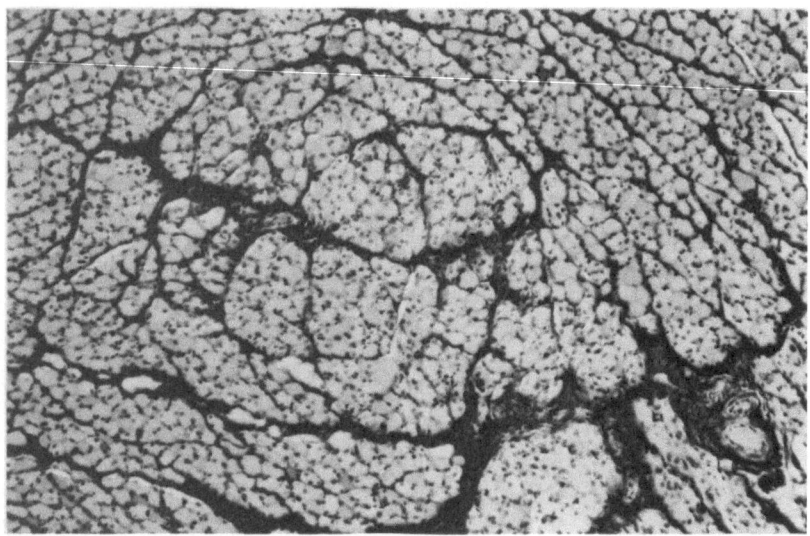

Fig. 45. Pseudolobular form of myoscleromatosis. TG V. 8th week. Van Gieson. Magn. ×40

The exact picture presented by a denervation atrophy depends on the extent of the deficit in nerve fibres resulting from stretching.

The hypertrophy of individual muscle fibres constitutes a genuine case of compensatory hypertrophy caused by the larger amount of work which has to be performed by those fibres which are still innervated. Regressive myopathic changes occurred only after fibres had grown beyond a certain "critical diameter".

The occurrence of central nuclei in more than 3 out of 100 muscle fibres is certainly pathological (Greenfield, Shy, Alvord, and Berg 1957). Although even in intact muscles the number of central nuclei increases in regions close to the tendon insertions (Adams, Denny-Brown, and Pearson 1962), this does not affect our conclusions because in our experiments we took tissue samples only from the muscle bellies.

The vacuolar degeneration observed by us probably corresponds to an earlier stage of the granular degeneration which is seen (Adams, Denny-Brown, and Pearson 1962).

The proliferation of sarcolemmal tissue with attendant appearance of pseudolobules, a myopathic appearance, resembles the myosclerotic form of Erb's dystrophy. Finding this appearance in association with a denervation atrophy is extraordinary because the proliferation of connective tissue which replaces destroyed muscle parenchyma begins after three to four months at the earliest.

Secondary myopathy is mainly due to disturbances of local circulation occurring in the areas affected by the denervation atrophy. There may be a connection between these disturbances and vascular innervation which is impaired both by the loss of nerve fibres and by continued mechanical irritation caused by nerve fibres left intact in the stretched nerve.

Scleromatosis is another pathogenetic factor determining the process of muscle fibre degeneration. The nutrient supply deteriorates because diffusion between capillaries and muscle cells is decisively interfered with.

However, myopathic changes accompanying denervation atrophies do not have any pathognomonic significance.

E. Synopsis of All Results
and Their Clinical Relevance

Part I

In human nerves repaired by end-to-end anastomosis under tension, injuries caused by stretching and especially by chronic strain of varying degrees cannot be clearly defined. As functional restitution is rarely complete even after tension-free suturing, a defect remaining in a nerve repaired under tension does not necessarily have to be a consequence of stretching alone. However, there is no way of determining clinically the extent to which the inadequate return of function in a nerve is explained solely by the strain.

The results of our animal experiments which involve several degrees of chronic nerve strain can be summed up as follows:

1. Mechanical properties of nerves

All peripheral nerves posses a certain amount of elasticity. There are individual differences in the Young's modulus (E) (the stress-strain ratio) of the sciatic nerves of rabbits, which ranges from 0.65 to 2.36 kp/mm². A low modulus means high elasticity, and vice versa. Also, there are individual variations in maximum elongation (ε), which varies between 5.9 and 16.5%; in tensile strength (σ_B), varying between 0.116 and 0.431 kp/mm²; and in the breaking force, which varies between 0.59 and 2.45 kp. These variations are due to the quality, quantity, and configuration of the tissue components which make up the nerve. Individual variations in the extensibility of nerves become increasingly evident as both tractive force and stress increase. Progressive elongation coincides with a reduction in the nerve's diameter and increasing stress, accompanied by a rise in intraneural pressure. Each degree of strain requires a different amount of tractive force and produces states of stress of varying intensity. Conversely, elongation rates vary between individuals subjected to the same amount of nerve stress and the same tractive force.

2. Mechanical resistance and behaviour under strain of the tissues involved

The resistance of the structural components of a nerve to stretching decreases in the following order: Epineurium, perineurium and endoneurium, vasa nervorum, axons and myelin sheaths. Large-calibre axons are more vulnerable than small-calibre ones.

Tensile strength is mainly dependent on the epineurium and peri-neurium. To a certain degree, the elastic properties of a nerve as a whole are preserved while its outer connective tissue sheaths are still intact. Unlike the outer tissue sheaths, the endoneurium's capacity for elongation is low; even lower still is the extensibility of the nerve fibres, which consist of viscous material. Demyelination attended by axonolysis occurs at strains as low as TG I, and rupture of axons from TG II onwards. The incidence of initial angiorrhexis and rupturing endoneurial sheaths increases with the elongation, and TG IV and V even result in transverse and longitudinal ruptures of the perineurium and epineurium.

3. Nature and extent of nerve lesions

All stages of strain entail parenchymal changes in proportion to their degree, the only exception being TG I, which in 8% of all cases produced no injury whatsoever. In all other cases, compression lesions occurred in the constricted area around the cylinder. The more extensive lesions produced by TG II—V are due to the combined influence of several mechanical factors:

a) Primary elongation;

b) a secondary increase in intraneural pressure caused by a reduc-tion of the nerve cross-section;

c) simultaneous stretching and compression of the vasa nervorum with its attendant disturbances of nutrient supply.

The most extensive losses of parenchyma always occur in those nerve segments which are subjected to the highest stress. As stress decreases proximally, the process of disintegration is confined to an increasing degree to the central nerve zones, which means, in fact, that the field of degeneration spreads conically through the trunk of the sciatic nerve. In some cases, which were observed only at TG I and II, degeneration spreads only unilaterally. Under TG IV and V, ruptures in the perineurium and epineurium led to external neural herniae. Distally, degeneration of the parenchyma is observed. The higher the degree of strain, the lower is the number of sciatic nerves left with a certain individually variable proportion of intact nerve fibres. The number of nerve fibres remaining unaffected is extremely small. The only exception is TG I, in which the proportion of the parenchyma left intact in a cross-section may actually be larger than the amount affected.

4. Ascent of the injury in the proximal portion of the nerve

In the proximal segment of the sciatic nerve, the centripetal spread of parenchymal degeneration depends on the degree of strain applied. The degeneration spreads more cranially as the tractive load imposed on the nerve increases.

The actual extent of spread varies within one and the same degree of strain because of individual differences in the elastic properties of the nerves.

From TG II onwards, compression phenomena begin to appear in the spinal roots at their passage through the intervertebral foramen which, to a stretched nerve, represents a bottleneck.

5. Individual variations in the consequences of stretching

Stretch injuries to the nerve caused by whatever degree of strain show individual variations. Differences may occur in

a) the proximal and distal extent of parenchymal changes;
b) the proximal and distal length of the ischaemic nerve segment;
c) the proportion of intact and injured nerve fibres;
d) the tensile strength especially of the outer connective tissue sheaths;
e) the history and intensity of degeneration and regeneration;
f) the degree of endoneurial fibrosis;
g) the extent to which spinal roots are affected by nerve stress;
h) the extent of retrograde changes in the nerve cells of the spinal ganglia and the anterior horns of the spinal cord.

6. History of the degeneration and regeneration of the parenchyma

The process of degeneration commences in zones of high stress and progresses proximally and distally through the sciatic nerve. The higher the degree of strain, the earlier will degeneration manifest itself (TG I: 3rd–7th day; from TG II onwards: first day). Axonolysis is generally completed by the end of the second week. The onset of axon regeneration is deferred even later as strain increases (TG I: 2nd week; TG V: 6th week). Axon regeneration is followed by restitution of the myelin sheaths at an interval of 1–2 weeks. During the later stages, the newly-formed remyelinated nerve fibres regain their natural undulation.

7. Impairment of the neural vascular network and of the nutrient supply

The increase in the endoneurial pressure level resulting from reduction of the nerve diameter causes the vasa nervorum to be compressed and stretched longitudinally. This, in turn, causes disturbances in the circulation and injuries due to ischaemia. Consequently, there is a secondary vascular as well as a primary mechanical causation of parenchymal injuries. The length of the ischaemic nerve segment depends on the degree of strain. Under TG II, it amounts to 7.8% of the total length of the nerve, increasing to 25.1% under TG V.

8. Retrograde cell reactions in the anterior columns of the spinal cord and in the spinal ganglia

The cellular changes which take place in motor neurons and sensory ganglia are identical with the phenomena of Nissl's central chromatolysis after neurotomy. Under TG I, only a small number of cell bodies show a delayed reaction, whereas the more extensive retrograde cellular involvement occurring at higher degrees of strain is obviously due to a greater proximal spread of the nerve lesion and to the considerably lower number of nerve fibres left intact. Restitution of the affected ganglion cells begins around the third week. In some cases, the process of alteration leads to cellular destruction, but this is not preponderant even with higher degrees of strain.

9. Types and extent of muscular affection

Initially, all degrees of sciatic nerve strain entail a generalized muscular atrophy. From the second week onwards, compensatory hypertrophy starts to develop in certain parts of the muscle which are still innervated. At the same time, patches of denervation atrophy begin to develop. Their spread depends on the degree of strain and thus on the extent of the nerve injury. Muscular involvement of this kind develops progressively, especially under higher degrees of strain. Hypertrophic muscle fibres undergo degenerative changes amounting to secondary non-specific myopathy. The atrophic muscle tissue undergoes sclerotic and lipomatous changes.

10. Clinical features

Under TG I, pain sensation and motor power disappeared in 20% of all cases, whereas they disappeared in the course of the first 5 days in 60% of all TG II cases, and from the first day in 100% of all TG III–V cases. Independently of the actual degree of nerve stretching, muscular atrophy varied widely, reaching its maximum around the 8th week. Neither is there a correlation between the intensity of stress acting on the sciatic nerve and the latent period before the manifestation of trophic lesions, their size, and their progress towards healing.

These results, which we obtained by animal experiments, can be applied to man only to a limited extent. Yet the elastic limits of human and rabbit sciatic nerves are approximately the same.

All our findings in connection with chronic nerve stretching are based on experiments within the elastic limit.

Part II

Our animal experiments were performed in order to determine the critical resection length as well as the critical gap distance of a nerve for direct end-to-end suturing.

The experimental results obtained by us from permanently stretched sciatic nerves in rabbits have shown the critical resection length to be 3% of the total nerve length, and the maximum permissible stress of direct end-to-end sutures to amount to 0.042 kp/mm².

Elongations as low as 4% (TG II) corresponding to a stress of 0.056 kp/mm² caused lesions in the proximal segment of all sciatic nerves analyzed which, however, in 32% of all cases extended only slightly beyond the theoretical suture in a centripetal direction. However, in 59% of all cases the proximal trunk of the sciatic nerve showed a lesion of 25 mm, and in 9% of all cases, of 50 mm. Consequently, the length of the lesions varies between 7.8 and 15.7% of the total nerve length and exceeds the critical resection length by a factor of 2.6 to 5.2. This clearly exceeds the limit of tolerable elongation or stress. In order to relate these results to human sciatic nerves, it is necessary to know the individual length of each nerve. Take, for example, the minimum (C) and the maximum (A) sciatic nerve length as determined from a number of human corpses: 91 cm (C) and 108 cm (A), corresponding to body lengths of 143 and 174 cm and to extremity lengths of 80 and 92 cm, respectively (ant. sup. iliac spine—ext. malleolus). Therefore, assuming a resection length of 4%, the ascent of the stretch injury after end-to-end suturing without the use of additional "manipulative" measures would be 7–14 cm (C) and 8–17 cm (A). After end-to-end union with the adjacent joints flexed, the stretch degeneration of the parenchyma would spread even further proximally as the mobility of the joint is restored by post-operative treatment. Unlike nerves repaired by tension-free end-to-end suturing the zone of axon regeneration of stretched nerves is not located at the end of the proximal nerve stump but at a higher level of the sciatic nerve trunk. Consequently, a relatively large part in the nerve must be re-innervated as far as its connexion to the effectors. As under a chronic elongation of 4% (TG II) axon regeneration commences as late as the 3rd week, and as the rate of axon growth of the pilot fibres is

3.28 mm/day, regeneration is delayed by 4–5 weeks as compared to tension-free nerve sutures. In human sciatic nerves, the delay would amount to 6–9 (C) and 6.5–10 weeks (A), respectively. This is the period required by the newly-formed nerve fibres to penetrate the stretch-injured proximal trunk of the sciatic nerve centrifugally and to reach the suture. Invasion of the distal nerve stump by sprouting axons may be impeded by a barrier of scar tissue which may have formed at the suture line in the meantime.

In human sciatic nerves, the critical resection length of 3% determined by us corresponds to 2.7 (C) and 3.2 cm (A). The absolute figures given by Forrester-Brown (1920), Babcock (1927), Highet and Holmes (1943), Grantham and Pollard (1951) are 2.5 to 5 times higher than ours (Table 1). We calculated that the figures given by these authors, expressed as a percentage of the total nerve length, are: Forrester-Brown (1920), 11% (C) and 9% (A); Babcock (1927), 15% (C) and 13% (A); Highet and Holmes (1943), 9% (C) and 8% (A); Grantham and Pollard (1951), 12% (C) and 10% (A). The extent of injury to the sciatic nerve caused by chronic elongations as low as 8 to 10% (TG IV and V), is illustrated by our animal experiments.

The critical resection lengths experimentally established by Highet and Sanders (1943), Denny-Brown and Doherty (1945), Liu, Benda, and Lewey (1948), Hoen and Brackett (1956), and Sunderland (1972), amounting to 6% and more, are also excessive. Millesi observed in 1972 that the functional recovery of sciatic nerves in rabbits after end-to-end anastomosis becomes problematic if more than 3% of the free nerve length is lost. This is the only finding which agrees with the results of our experiments.

In nerve injuries, the absolute defect consists of the traumatic loss of substance and the tissue deficit caused by sufficient surgical freshening of the nerve stumps. This defect must not exceed 3%, which corresponds to the critical resection length. Moreover, the nerve gap is increased further by the retraction of the nerve ends, which means that critical gap distance and critical resection length are not the same. Severing 16 healthy rabbit sciatic nerves resulted in gaps of 6.6 ± 1.5 mm with the extremity flexed, and of 15.5 ± 2.5 mm with the extremity straightened out. These figures correspond to an average of 2 to 5% of the total nerve length. Together with the critical resection length of 3%, the retraction sizes thus determined add up to critical gap distances of 5–8%. In human sciatic nerves, the critical gap distance would be 4.6–7.3 cm (C) and 5.4–8.6 cm (A) in nerves of 91 cm (C) and 108 cm (A). As the critical gap distance is highly dependant on the posture of the joints, when operating on peripheral nerves, the position of the extremity must be taken into account. This cannot be applied to nerve injuries with complete division especially when secondarily repaired, for we can assume that in the meantime the nerve stumps have retracted to a maximum and are fixed by scar tissue because of the extent of movements of the limb. Obviously we find the same situation when there is an accompanying fracture of the bone with abnormal movement of the extremity.

In such cases the critical gap distance always amounts practically to 8%. As there are other factors which influence the extent of the retraction (Chapter A) this helps to explain the variations which are found.

After the resection of a 16 cm fibrosarcoma from a human sciatic nerve, Petrov and Solarov (1965) observed that the gap increased by 4 cm. After neurotomy of a normal rabbit sciatic nerve, Millesi (1973) reported a gap of 8–12 mm, and Koschitz-Kosic (1960) reported a retraction of up to 40 mm in the sciatic nerves of young dogs. We demonstrated that, after chronic stretching of 1–4 weeks, the nerve gap of a stretched nerve, unlike that of a normal nerve, amounts to a mere 4.2 ± 1.5 mm after being severed with the joints flexed, independently of the degree of strain applied. This reduction in retractility is obviously due to a change in the elastic properties of the nerve which is caused by stretch injuries. Retractility increases again from the 4th week onwards.

Critical resection length varies according to individual variations in the extensibility of nerves and in the extent to which the lesion of the parenchyma spreads proximally. However, in practical neurosurgery there is no way of determining the mechanical characteristics of the nerves of each patient individually. Therefore, the lowest figures from the entire range of individual variations must be assumed to constitute the limit, and each resection length and elongation exceeding this limit must be regarded as hazardous. One of the main factors limiting critical resection length to 3% of the total nerve length is the fact that ruptures of axons occur proximally and distally from the theoretical suture-line from TG II (4%) onwards. Additional factors are histological changes in the structure of the nerve roots, and retrograde reactions in the parent cell bodies of the anterior horns and spinal ganglia.

If one oversteps the critical resection length of 3% and the critical gap distance of 5–8% there is no room for manoeuvre to approximate the ends and allow suture of the nerve without tension. Consequently both nerve and suture are subjected to increased stress which causes stretch injuries to the nerve. Considering that the primary injury alone will lead to retrograde degeneration involving partial destruction of the ganglion cells, and that any secondary suture is bound to cause a second lesion in the proximal stump because of undermining and freshening, which means a renewal of nerve cell changes, any additional stretching caused by tension on the suture is bound to increase the injury to the parenchyma even further. Even after a tension-free suture performed 3 or even 6 months after an injury, the distal nerve segment shows a reduced number of regenerating fibres whose diameter, growth rate and maturation are reduced (Sanders and Young 1944). If a delayed secondary suture is made under stress, the process of recovery already not very effective is compromised even further, so that the prognosis is not at all good. The same applies to high-level nerve injuries, whose prospects of effective regeneration are low in any case. The more proximal the site of a lesion, the more adversely its chances of recovery will be affected by any additional though moderate stress on the suture.

Extensive nerve defects, which do not permit adapting the nerve ends during initial debridement, are sometimes treated by fixing the nerve stumps to their bed under "slight" tension to reduce retraction and shrinkage until an early secondary suture can be made. Even in those cases, elongation must not go beyond the critical limit. Moreover, the success of secondary anastomosis would be jeopardized by the application of any lengthening procedures involving the gradual stretching of nerve stumps to bridge a gap which it was impossible to close during primary debridement. This applies in any case, no matter which of the following methods is used: Bethe (1916), Müller (1917), Baron and Schreiber (1918), Hoen (1948), or Hoen and Brackett (1956). At this juncture, we would like to mention the method proposed by Seifert (1972) which is based on Wagner's (1971) operation of gaining extra length by osteotomy in the lower extremity which also involves elongating the nerve. This procedure yields a daily increase in nerve length of 1.5 mm. Although, in this case, the maximum elongation of the nerve is still within the limit of tolerance (0.2%/day), the interval required for each lengthening is too long for an injured and severed nerve. A neuroma might develop in the meantime, and its unavoidable resection would mean another nerve defect.

Although critical resection length and maximum permissible limit of elongation have been determined to be as high as 3%, lesions of the nerve may be caused by a permanent stretching as little as 2%. A 2% nerve elongation (TG I) involves a mechanical stress of $0.028 \, kp/mm^2$, which is enough to cause compression damage to the nerve loop around the cylinder. This damage occurs in 92% of all cases. However, as it affects mainly the nerve loop, i.e., the segment of nerve the resection of which is simulated, in general this finding is not clinically relevant to the phenomenon of critical resection length. In 16% of all cases, we observed an ascent of the degeneration process. We cannot entirely exclude the possibility of this being wholly or partially due to stress. In the long run, nerves will not tolerate any curtailing of their physiological range of extensibility, even in a limited way.

The fact that stretch injuries occur at elongations as low as 2% is due to individual variations in the elastic properties of nerves as well as to the pathogenic significance of the anatomy of the nerve and to the time factor. The topography of peripheral nerves shows that in some cases they have to pass through physiological or pathological constrictions which are comparable to those caused by the cylinders used in our animal experiments. In all cases of resection lengths of 2% and more, therefore, compression injuries are likely to occur if a nerve is directly sutured end-to-end on a level with or in the close neighbourhood of a bottleneck. The nerve is stretched and pressed onto its support just like the strings of a violin passing over the bridge.

Therefore, it is virtually impossible to avoid compression lesions when repairing by end-to-end suture a defect in the radial nerve of up to 2% of the total nerve length, if the lesion is located in the area around the shaft of the humerus where the nerve runs through the sulcus and is in direct contact with the periosteum. Permanent compression of this kind is bound to affect the process of nerve regeneration adversely. Should the resection be longer than 2%, the effect of compression will be enhanced in proportion and supplemented by changes due to stretching. For this reason, the critical resection length pertaining to end-to-end sutures applied close to where the nerve passes through a confined space is not 3 but 2% if it is impossible to circumvent or to remove the constriction (*e.g.*, by volar transposition of the ulnar nerve in the elbow region, by excision of an exostosis etc.).

If a nerve defect is longer than the critical resection length determined by us (3% generally, and 2% in the neighbourhood of constrictions), and if the critical gap distance amounts to more than 5–8% of the total nerve length, the only alternative method for reconstructing a nerve is autografting. It is still said rather often that autografting is indicated only if tension-free neurorrhaphy is impossible in spite of "manipulative" auxiliary measures, such as mobilization, transposition, and flexing of joints (Bunnell and Boyes 1939, Brooks 1955, 1972, Nigst 1962, Mumenthaler and Schliack 1965). Autografting is not an emergency solution to be tried only after direct end-to-end suture has failed. In this instance the more or less extensive mobilization and transposition of the nerve as well as the danger of mechanical damage as a result of the extreme flexion of the adjacent joints and the insufficient blood circulation in the vessels of the nerve, severely prejudice the chances of clinical success for autografting. Ischaemia in the isolated nerve stumps causes fibrosis not only in the stumps but in the graft as well, thus impeding the process of regeneration and possibly even causing it to turn neuromatous (Schröder and Seiffert 1970). In the case of an injury to the ulnar nerve in the forearm, Klar (1943), for instance, prefers autografting even to transposing the nerve to the anterior aspect of the internal condyle.

Using the supporting measures traditionally associated with the repair of a nerve injury, such as flexing neighbouring joints for relief of tension, is not really justifiable any more in modern neurosurgery. It can be taken for granted that even the cautious and gradual mobilization of a joint after an operation will cause stretch injuries to a nerve with a tension-free primary suture (Baron and Schreiber 1918, Stookey 1922, Küttner 1931, Dumas 1940, Leriche 1940, Highet and Holmes 1943, Highet and Sanders 1943, Spurling 1945, Thomson, Ritchie, French, and Wrork 1946, Woodhall 1959, Millesi 1972, Sunderland 1972, Samii 1973). Moreover, mobilization and transposition of a nerve are justified only if they are not too extensive and do not involve flexing of the joints; the surgeon has to be reasonably sure before using these methods that a subsequent direct tension-free union will be possible. This is the case only in certain nerves whose topography in the area of the lesion is suitable. For instance, a defect in the ulnar nerve at the level of the elbow joint can be closed by anterior transposition in such a fashion that even gap sizes of more than 5 to 8% can be bridged without autografting and without tension. If these conditions do not apply, autografting is indicated, especially so as the functional results of this procedure have benefited considerably from the introduction of the surgical microscope and of the perineurial interfascicular suturing technique (Edshage 1964, Michon and Masse 1964, Smith 1964, Millesi, Ganglberger, and Berger 1966, 1967, Millesi 1968, 1969, 1972, Geldmacher 1969, Michon 1969, Samii and Willebrand 1970, Maxion, Samii, Scheinpflug, and Wallenborn 1972, Samii, Schürmann, Wallenborn, and Scheinpflug 1972, Samii and Wallenborn 1972, Samii 1975, Pia et al. 1978).

The best possible materials for use in autografting are freshly resected cutaneous nerves. It is obvious that interfascicular anastomosis is possible only in nerves whose cross-sectional arrangement of fascicles is similar. Anyhow, it is not always possible to rejoin identical proximal and distal segments in a pedicle graft. Even interfascicular surgery cannot ensure the anatomically perfect reconstitution of a nerve, because fascicular patterns change constantly over its entire course. Despite this imperfection, there is a good prospect of a large proportion of the sprouting axons getting into proper alignment peripherally when the fascicles of the quasi-congruent nerve quadrants are joined together.

The factors which have improved the results of interfascicular autoplasty and microsurgery are: Tissue is preserved to a maximum degree; the extent of the nerve lesion can be reliably ascertained; nerve stumps can be freshened extensively; total resection of the epineurium, which is the basis of fibrous reaction especially in the suture zone; exact approximation of the nerve ends with suturing free from tension; nutritional damage is avoided by the use of small calibre cutaneous nerves; any Schwann's cells surviving in the graft are preserved, and the transplant has no antigenic potential. These factors are confirmed by clinical and experimental studies performed so far by Millesi (1972, 1976), Buck-Gramcko (1972), Samii and Kahl (1972), Samii and Wallenborn (1972), Maxion, Samii, Scheinpflug, and Wallenborn (1972), and Samii (1975). According to these facts, nerve defects in excess of the critical resection length for end-to-end sutures can be successfully bridged by interfascicular transplantation of cable grafts. Prognosis depends on the time which has elapsed since the occurrence of the injury, the level of the lesion, the state of the nerve bed, the age of the patient, and especially on the length of the graft. The length of pedicle grafts must always be somewhat in excess of requirements to allow for shrinkage after resection and transplantation. Authors are not in agreement on the surplus length required compared to the actual size of the lesion, the figures given by the following authors ranging from 12 to 25% (Seddon 1963, Petrov and Solarov 1966, Maurer 1971, Brooks 1972).

As there is a distinct drop in the speed of axon growth in the graft (Gutmann and Sanders 1942, 1943) an endoneurial and perineurial barrier of scar tissue may have formed at the distal suture line before the axons can reach it. If grafts exceeding 2.5 or 3 cm in length had to be transplanted according to the traditional method, secondary debridement was required to resect the peripheral suture zone, and the nerve had to be re-sutured to re-start the process of axon growth which had come to a standstill (Lewis 1923, Davis and Cleveland 1934, Dogliotti 1938, Röttgen 1949, 1959, Bsteh 1953, Bsteh and Millesi 1960, Millesi 1968, 1969). Modern surgical technique requires secondary debridement only if the length of the transplant is between 5 and 20 cm (Millesi 1969, 1972). Impediments to axon growth of this kind limit the effectiveness even of autografting, which means that we have to differentiate between the critical resection length of end-to-end suturing and that of autografting.

F. Summary

One of the essential problems involved in the surgical debridement of nerve injuries is the bridging of tissue defects. At present, two major methods of reconstituting the nerve are in general use: Direct end-to-end suturing of nerve stumps, and autografting.

Considering the pros and cons of each method, the problem which comes to mind is the question concerning their respective indication.

Critical resection length has hitherto been synonymous with the maximum length of a defect which it was still possible to repair by a direct end-to-end suture, using "manipulative" measures such as flexing of the neighbouring joints, mobilization, and transposition of the nerve. The figures given in the literature as representing the critical resection length vary somewhat; according to our clinical experience, all these figures are too high, the limiting factor being not the distance to be bridged but the amount of nerve strain and stress involved. For this reason, it is especially important as far as end-to-end suturing is concerned to determine the exact maximum defect length at which this method guarantees the functionally successful reconstruction of a nerve without any damage due to stretching and without the use of any "manipulative" measures.

Five groups comprising a total of 56 adult rabbits were subjected to unilateral stretching of the sciatic nerve, elongations of 2, 4, 6, 8, and 10⁰/₀ of the total length of the nerve being permanently maintained over periods of time ranging from 1 day to a maximum of 35 weeks. The five degrees of strain described above corresponded to fictitious resection lengths and nerve gaps of the same dimension. We stretched intact nerves so as to avoid any disguising of the results by a parenchymal degeneration due to neurotomy. The test procedure used and specifically developed for this purpose adequately reproduced the behaviour of a nerve under strain after end-to-end union. For this reason, the method employed by us was exceptionally well suited to the purpose of our study, which was to determine anew the exact extent of the critical resection length.

Our morphological findings show that nerve lesions will occur at all degrees of strain even before the elastic limit is reached. The extent and proximal spread of parenchymal affection increased in direct proportion to the tractive force. However, the extent of injury produced by one and the same degree of strain varied from one individual to another, depending on the elastic properties of each nerve.

Elongation by 2% caused local compression lesions in constricted sections of the nerve, indicating that the physiological range of extensibility of the nerve had been curtailed. Elongations between 4 and 10% produced more extensive nerve lesions; these resulted from the coincidence of several factors: a) primary longitudinal stretching; b) a secondary increase in intraneural pressure due to a reduction of the nerve cross-section; c) simultaneous stretching and compression of the vasa nervorum, which causes a deficiency in the nutrient supply. At elongations of 4–10%, compression phenomena were observed in the spinal roots at their passage through the inter-vertebral foramen which acted on the stretched nerve as a bottleneck. Retrograde cellular reactions occurred in the spinal cord. Compared to neurotomy, axon regeneration was delayed, the period which elapsed before its onset increasing nearly in direct proportion to the degree of strain applied. During the later stages, fibre undulation reconstituted itself, which seemed to indicate that the state of chronic stretching had been overcome.

By analysis of our findings, we established the critical resection length for end-to-end suturing of pheripheral nerves as 3% of the total length of the nerve, and the maximum permissible stress as 0.042 kp/mm². Even permanent stretching of 4% clearly went beyond the limit of tolerable elongation. Therefore, as soon as the resection length exceeds 3%, the free scope of the nerve, which is the only factor permitting a tension-free suture, is exhausted. The increased stress then acting on both the nerve and the suture line causes stretch injuries.

Due to the compression injuries observed at an elongation of 2%, the critical resection length for end-to-end sutures is limited to that figure if the suture is located either at the level or in the close neigh-bourhood of anatomical or pathological bottlenecks.

Critical resection length is defined as the length of a limited nerve segment to be severed from a continuous nerve trunk. It does not incorporate the effect of nerve end retraction. The critical gap distance does incorporate the effect of retraction both after a trauma and after resection. It represents the sum total of the critical resection length and the extent of retraction. As the latter differs, the critical gap distance may range from 5 to 8%. In practice however, the critical gap distance most commonly amounts to 8%.

The results obtained from our experiments show that an end-to-end suture not involving the application of any "manipulative" auxiliary measures is indicated whenever the absolute nerve gap to be closed does not extend beyond 5 to 8% of the total nerve length. If, however, an analysis of the case shows that the resection length exceeds the critical value of 3% (2% close to a nerve's passage through a bottleneck), or that the gap size exceeds the critical limit of 5 to 8%, the only procedure indicated for the reconstruction of the nerve is interfascicular autografting.

References   82

Adams, R. W., Denny-Brown, D., Pearson, C. M.: Diseases of muscle. 2nd edition.
New York: P. Hoeber. 1962.
Alexander, E. Jr., Woods, R. P., Weiss, P.: Further experiments on bridging of
long nerve gaps in monkeys. Proc. Soc. exp. Biol. Med. *68* (1948), 380—382.
Babcock, W. W.: A standard technique for operations on peripheral nerves with
special reference to the closure of large gaps. Surg. Gynec. Obstet. *45* (1927),
364—378.
Baron, A., Schreiber, W.: Über die direkte Nervenvereinigung bei großen Nerven-
defekten. Münch. med. Wschr. *65* (1918), 446—449.
Bethe, A.: Allgemeine Anatomie und Physiologie des Nervensystems. Leipzig:
Thieme. 1903.
— Zwei neue Methoden der Überbrückung größerer Nervenlücken. Dtsch. med.
Wschr. *42* (1916), 1311—1314.
— Die Haltbarkeit von Nervennähten und -narben und die Spannungsverhältnisse
gedehnter Nerven. Dtsch. med. Wschr. *42* (1916), 1277—1311.
Bielschowsky, M.: Über das Verhalten der Achsenzylinder in Geschwülsten des
Nervensystems und in Kompressionsgebieten des Rückenmarks. J. Psychol.
Neurol. (Leipzig) *7* (1906), 101—139.
— Unger, E.: Überbrückung großer Nervenlücken; Beiträge zur Kenntnis der
Degeneration und Regeneration peripherer Nerven. J. Psychol. Neurol. (Leipzig)
22 (1917), 267—318.
Björkesten, G. af: Über Nervenverletzungen im Finnisch-Russischen Kriege 1939
bis 1940. Zbl. Neurochir. *6* (1941), 107—113.
— Suture of war injuries to peripheral nerves: clinical studies of results. Acta
chir. scand. *95*, Suppl. 119 (1947).
— Clinical experiences with nerve grafting. J. Neurosurg. *5* (1948), 450—463.
— Nervennaht: Indikationen, Technik und Ergebnisse. Melsunger Med. Mitt. *46*,
Heft 116 (1972), 141—147.
Blum, A.: De l'élongation des nerfs. Arch. génér. de méd. *1*, (1878), 22—36.
Brecht, K.: Muskelphysiologie. In: Lehrbuch der Physiologie. Ed. by Keidel, v.,
W. D. Stuttgart: Thieme. 1967.
Brooks, D.: The place of nerve-grafting in orthopaedic surgery. J. Bone Jt Surg.
37 A (1955), 299—304.
— Diskussionsbemerkung. Symposium über Verletzungen peripherer Nerven.
Kassel-Wilhelmshöhe, 3.—4. 2. 1972. Melsunger Med. Mitt. *46*, Heft 116
(1972), 160.
— Autogene Nerventransplantate zur Überbrückung großer Defekte. Symposium
über Verletzungen peripherer Nerven. Kassel-Wilhelmshöhe, 3.—4. 2. 1972.
Melsunger Med. Mitt. *46*, Heft 116 (1972), 179—180.
Bsteh, F. X.: Experimentelles zur Frage der zweizeitigen Nerveninterplantation.
Zbl. Neurochir *13* (1953), 23—28.
— Millesi, H.: Zur Kenntnis der zweizeitigen Nerveninterplantation bei ausge-
dehntem peripherem Nervendefekt. Klin. Med. *15* (1960), 571—578.
Buck-Gramcko, D.: Wiederherstellung durchtrennter peripherer Nerven. Chir.
Praxis *15* (1971), 55—63.

Buck-Gramcko, D.: Diskussionsbemerkung. Symposium über Verletzungen peripherer Nerven. Kassel-Wilhelmshöhe, 3.—4. 2. 1972. Melsunger Med. Mitt. 46, Heft 116 (1972), 154, 156, 205.

Bunnell, S., Boyes, J. H.: Nerve grafts. Amer. J. Surg. 44 (1939), 64—75.

Cajal, R. y. S.: Variaciones morfologicas, normales y patologicas del reticulo neurofibrilar. Trab. Lab. Invest. biol. (Madrid) 3 (1904), 9—15.

Causey, G.: The functional importance of the blood supply of peripheral nerves. Ann. roy. Coll. Surg. Engl. 16 (1955), 267—383.

Chao, Y. C., Tsang, Y. C., Tsui, C. T.: Nerve regeneration through a gap. An experimental study. Chin. med. J. 81 (1962), 740—748.

Conrad, T.: Experimentelle Untersuchungen über Nervendehnung. Inaug. Dissertation, Greifswald 1876.

Cutler, E. C., Gross, R. E.: The surgical treatment of tumours of the peripheral nerves. Ann. Surg. 104 (1936), 436—452.

Darkschewitsch, L.: Die pathologische Anatomie der Muskeln. In: Handbuch der pathologischen Anatomie, Nervensystem, ed. by Flatau, Jacobsohn, and Minor. Berlin: Karger. 1904.

Davis, L., Cleveland, D.: Experimental studies in nerve transplants. Ann. Surg. 99 (1934), 271—283.

Debove et Laborde: Recherches sur la détermination expérimentale des effets de l'élongation des nerfs, et du mécanisme de ces effets dans l'état pathologique et dans l'état physiologique. Gaz. méd. Paris 3 (1881), 96—97.

Denny-Brown, D., Doherty, M. M.: Effects of transient stretching of peripheral nerves. Arch. Neurol. Psychiat. (Chic.) 54 (1945), 116—129.

Dogliotti, A. M.: I processi riparativi delle lesioni dei nervi periferici. VIII. Kongr. f. Unfallmed. 2 (1938), 419.

Dumas, R.: Blessures des nerfs; résultats éloignés du traitement chirurgical et indications opératoires. Presse méd. 48 (1940), 99—101.

Duncan, D.: Alterations in the structure of nerves caused by restricting their growth with ligatures. J. Neuropath. exp. Neurol. 7 (1948), 261—273.

Durante, G.: Anatomie pathologique des muscles. In: Manuel d'histologie pathologique, ed. by Cornil and Ranvier, Paris 1902.

Duschek, A.: Vorlesungen über höhere Mathematik, Bd. II, S. 147—150. Wien: Springer. 1963.

Edshage, S.: Peripheral nerve suture. A technique for improved intraneural topography evaluation of some suture materials. Acta chir. scand., Suppl. 331 (1964), 1—104.

— Peripheral nerve injuries. Diagnosis and treatment. New Engl. J. Med. 278 (1968), 1431—1436.

Eicke, W. J.: Die Hallervorden-Spatzsche Krankheit. In: Handbuch der speziellen pathologischen Anatomie und Histologie, ed. by Henke-Lubarsch, Bd. XIII/1 A, S. 845. Berlin-Göttingen-Heidelberg: Springer. 1957.

Fazekas, I. Gy., Kósa, F., Szendrényi, J., Jobba, Gy., Bajnóczky, I.: Zerreißfestigkeit der proximalen Nervenstämme der unteren Extremität. Z. Rechtsmed. 70 (1972), 178—183.

— — — — —: Die Zerreißfestigkeit der Nervenstämme der oberen Extremität. Z. Rechtsmed. 70 (1972), 229—234.

Forrester-Brown, M.: Difficulties in the diagnosis of nerve function. Brit. J. Surg. 7 (1920), 495—501.

— The possibilities of suture after extensive nerve injury. J. orthop. Surg. 3 (1921), 277—287.

Friede, R. L., Samorajski, T.: Relation between the number of myelin lamellae and axon circumference in fibers of vagus and sciatic nerves of mice. J. comp. Neurol. *130* (1967), 223—232.

Geldmacher, J.: Ergebnisse nach Naht peripherer Nerven an den oberen Extremitäten. Mschr. Unfallheilk. *68* (1965), 308—313.

— Die Wiederherstellung verletzter Nerven. Münch. med. Wschr. *111* (1969), 2675—2679.

Gerhardt, U.: Das Kaninchen. Leipzig: Klinkhardt. 1909.

Gilette: Elongation des nerfs. Gaz. des hôpit. 1880, p. 1197.

Glees, P.: Observations on the structure of the connective tissue sheaths of cutaneous nerves. J. Anat. (Lond.) *77* (1943), 153—159.

Grantham, E. G., Pollard, C.: Peripheral nerve surgery. Ann. Surg. *134*, (1951), 145—150.

Greenfield, J. G., Shy, G. M., Alvord, E. E., Berg, L.: An atlas of muscle pathology in neuromuscular disease. Edinburgh-London: Livingstone. 1957.

Gutmann, E.: Die funktionelle Regeneration der peripheren Nerven. Berlin: Akademie-Verlag. 1958.

— Kucerova, M.: Vestnik Cs. zool. spol. *11* (1947), 145; cited by Gutmann, E., 1958.

— Sanders, F. K.: Functional recovery following nerve grafts and other types of nerve bridging. Brain *65* (1942), 373—408.

— Recovery of fibre numbers and diameters in the regeneration of peripheral nerves. J. Physiol. (Lond.) *101* (1943), 489—518.

Haftek, J.: Stretch injury of peripheral nerve. J. Bone Jt Surg. *52 B* (1970), 354—365.

Hager, H.: Regenerationsvorgänge am Neuron des zentralen Nervensystems. Verh. dtsch. Ges. Path. *50* (1966), 255—275.

— Allgemeine morphologische Pathologie des Nervengewebes. In: Handbuch der allgemeinen Pathologie, Bd. III/3. Ed. by Altmann, H.-W., Büchner, F., Cottier, H., Holle, G., Letterer, E., Masshoff, W., Meessen, H., Roulet, F., Seifert, G., Siebert, G., Studer, A. Berlin-Heidelberg-New York: Springer. 1968.

Hanefeld, F.: Histochemisch nachweisbare Veränderungen im Enzymmuster des Nerven nach experimenteller Durchtrennung. Dtsch. Z. Nervenheilk. *188* (1966), 357—383.

Hartung, G., Arnold, G.: Histomechanische Eigenschaften peripherer Nerven. Nervenarzt *44* (1973), 80—84.

Heidenhain, M.: Plasma und Zelle. Eine allgemeine Anatomie der lebendigen Masse. Jena: G. Fischer. 1911.

Heller, I. H., Wolfe, L. S., Hesse, S.: Studies on the metabolic effects of a substance found in peripheral nerves. J. Neurochem. *9* (1962), 443—449.

Highet, W. B., Holmes, W.: Traction injuries to lateral popliteal nerves and traction injuries to peripheral nerves after suture. Brit. J. Surg. *30* (1943), 212—233.

— Sanders, F. K.: The effects of stretching nerves after suture. Brit. J. Surg. *30* (1943), 355—369.

Hoen, T. I.: The repair of peripheral nerve lesions. Amer. J. Surg. *72* (1946), 489—495.

— Bridging of nerve gaps by lengthening of central end. Arch. Neurol. Psychiat. (Chic.) *60* (1948), 543—545.

— Brackett, C. E.: Peripheral nerve lengthening. I. Experimental. J. Neurosurg. *13* (1956), 43—62.

Holmes, W., Young, J. Z.: Nerve regeneration after immediate and delayed suture. J. Anat. (Lond.) *77* (1942), 63—96.

Ihering, v.: Das periphere Nervensystem der Wirbeltiere. Leipzig: Vogel. 1878.

Jacob, H.: Sekundäre, retrograde und transsynaptische Degeneration. In: Handbuch der speziellen pathologischen Anatomie und Histologie, ed. by Henke-Lubarsch, Bd. XIII/1 A, S. 301. Berlin-Göttingen-Heidelberg: Springer. 1957.

Jamin, F.: Experimentelle Untersuchungen zur Lehre von der Atrophie gelähmter Muskeln. Habil.-Schrift, Erlangen 1904.

— Degeneration und Regeneration. Transplantation. Hypertrophie und Atrophie. Myositis. In: Handbuch der normalen und pathologischen Physiologie, Bd. XIII/1. Berlin: Springer. 1925.

Kirschner, M.: Zur Behandlung großer Nervendefekte. Dtsch. med. Wschr. *43* (1917), 739—747.

Klar, E.: Über Erfahrungen und Erfolge bei Anwendung der plastischen Überbrückung von Defekten in peripheren Nerven. Z. ges. Neurol. Psychiat. *176* (1943), 533—555.

Koch, E.: Über den Einfluß vorübergehender Blutabsperrung auf den Längsquerschnittstrom des Warmblüternerven. Z. ges. exp. Med. *50* (1926), 238—257.

Kohlrausch, F.: Praktische Physik, Bd. I, pp. 45—50. Stuttgart: Teubner. 1968.

Koschitz-Kosic, H.: Chirurgie und Regeneration durchtrennter peripherer Nerven, S. 37. Berlin: VEB Volk und Gesundheit. 1960.

Krause, W.: Die Anatomie des Kaninchens in topographischer und operativer Rücksicht. Leipzig: W. Engelmann. 1884.

Krenkel, W.: Indikationen zur operativen Behandlung peripherer Nerven. Symposium über Verletzungen peripherer Nerven. Kassel-Wilhelmshöhe, 3.—4. 2. 1972. Melsunger Med. Mitt. *46*, Heft 116 (1972), 127—140.

Kreutzberg, G. W.: Lokalisierter Oxydoreduktasenanstieg bei der Wallerschen Degeneration des peripheren Nerven. Naturwissensch. *50* (1963), 96.

— Enzymhistochemische Veränderungen in Axonen des Rückenmarks nach Durchschneidung der langen Bahnen. Dtsch. Z. Nervenheilk. *185* (1963), 308—318.

— Changes of coenzyme (TPN) diaphorase and TPN-linked dehydrogenase during axonal reaction of the nerve cell. Nature (Lond.) *199* (1963), 393—394.

— Allgemeine Pathologie der Nervenverletzungen. In: Neuro-Traumatologie, Bd. II. Ed. by Kessel, F. K., Gutmann, L., Maurer, G. München-Berlin-Wien: Urban & Schwarzenberg. 1971.

Krücke, W.: Erkrankungen des peripheren Nervensystems. In: Handbuch der speziellen pathologischen Anatomie und Histologie, Bd. XIII/5, ed. by Lubarsch, O., Henke, F., Rössle, R., Scholz, W. Berlin-Göttingen-Heidelberg: Springer. 1955.

— Diskussionsbemerkung. Symposium über Verletzungen peripherer Nerven. Kassel-Wilhelmshöhe, 3.—4. 2. 1972. Melsunger Med. Mitt. *46*, Heft 116 (1972), 365.

— Pathologie der peripheren Nerven. In: Handbuch der Neurochirurgie, Bd. VII/3. Ed. by Olivecrona, H., Tönnis, W., Krenkel, W. Berlin-Heidelberg-New York: Springer. 1974.

Küttner, H.: Die Chirurgie der peripheren Nerven. Arch. klin. Chir. *167* (1931), 263—284.

Leriche, R.: De la vie végétative des nerfs périphériques d'après l'observation chirurgicale. Presse méd. *1* (1941), 641—645.

— Des causes d'échéc des sutures nerveuses; moyens d'y pallier. Presse méd. *1* (1940), 345—348.

Lewis, D.: Boston med. Surg. 1923, p. 188; cited by Millesi, H., 1968.

Liu, C. T., Benda, C. E., Lewey, F. H.: Tensile strength of human nerves. Arch. Neurol. Psychiat. (Chic.) *59* (1948), 322—336.

Löbker, K.: Über die Kontinuitätsresektion der Knochen behufs Ausführung sekundärer Sehnen- und Nervennaht. Zbl. Chir. *11* (1884), 841—845.

Lorenz, H.: Die Muskelerkrankung. In: Handbuch der speziellen pathologischen Therapie innerer Krankheiten, Bd. XI. Jena: Fischer. 1904.

Lundborg, G., Rydevik, B.: Effects of stretching the tibial nerve of the rabbit. J. Bone Jt Surg. *55 B* (1973), 390—401.

Mackenzie, I. G., Woods, C. G.: Causes of failure after repair of the median nerve. J. Bone Jt Surg. *43 B* (1961), 465—473.

Marcus et Wiet: Elongation des pneumogastriques. Glycosurie provoquée par l'elongation des deux sciatiques. Gaz. des hôpit. 1881, pp. 477—478.

Maurer, G.: Klinik und Therapie der Verletzungen der peripheren Nerven. In: Neuro-Traumatologie II., ed. by Kessel, F. K., Gutmann, L., Maurer, G. München-Berlin-Wien: Urban & Schwarzenberg. 1971.

Maxion, H., Samii, M. Scheinpflug, W., Wallenborn, R.: Elektromyographische Verlaufsuntersuchungen nach Nervennaht und Nerventransplantation beim Kaninchen. Z. EEG-EMG *3* (1972), 89—94.

McQuillan, W. M.: Origin of fibrosis after peripheral nerve division. Lancet *2* (1965), 1220.

Mellick, R. S., Cavanach, J. B.: Longitudinal movement of radioiodinated albumin within extravascular spaces of peripheral nerves following three systems of experimental trauma. J. Neurol. Neurosurg. Psychiat. (Lond.) *30* (1967), 458—463.

— Changes in blood vessel permeability during degeneration and regeneration in peripheral nerves. Brain *91* (1968), 141—160.

Meyenburg, H. v.: Die quergestreifte Muskulatur. In: Handbuch der speziellen pathologischen Anatomie und Histologie, ed. by Henke-Lubarsch. Bd. IX/1. Berlin: Springer. 1929.

Michon, J.: Die Nervennaht unter dem Mikroskop. Handchirurgie *1* (1969), 75—76.

— Masse, P.: Der optimale Zeitpunkt für die Nervennaht bei Verletzungen der oberen Extremität. Rev. Chir. orthop. *50* (1964), 205—212.

Millesi, H.: Klinische und experimentelle Erfahrungen bei der Wiederherstellung peripherer Nervenläsion. Langenbecks Arch. klin. Chir. *301* (1962), 893—897.

— Zum Problem der Überbrückung von Defekten peripherer Nerven. Wien. med. Wschr. *9/10* (1968), 182—187.

— Wiederherstellung durchtrennter peripherer Nerven und Nerventransplantation. Münch. med. Wschr. *111* (1969), 2669—2674.

— Diskussionsbemerkung. Symposium über Verletzungen peripherer Nerven. Kassel-Wilhelmshöhe, 3.—4. 2. 1972. Melsunger med. Mitt. *46*, Heft 116 (1972), 153.

— Indikation und Technik der autologen und interfaszikulären Nerventransplantation. Symposium über Verletzungen peripherer Nerven. Kassel-Wilhelmshöhe, 3.—4. 2. 1972. Melsunger med. Mitt. *46*, Heft 116 (1972), 181—188.

— Diskussion über Ergebnisse der interfaszikulären autologen Nerventransplantation. Symposium über Verletzungen peripherer Nerven. Kassel-Wilhelmshöhe, 3.—4. 2. 1972. Melsunger med. Mitt. *46*, Heft 116 (1972), 203—204.

— Ref.: Selecta 1973, Nr. *4*, 246.

— Moderne Behandlung von Nervenverletzungen. Zbl. Neurochir. *37* (1976), 210—211.

Millesi, H., Ganglberger, J., Berger, A.: Vortrag in der Sitzung der Gesellschaft der Ärzte in Wien, 18. 11. 1966.
— Erfahrungen mit der Mikrochirurgie peripherer Nerven. Chir. plast. reconstr. 3 (1967), 47—55.
Müller, E.: Über die Ausnützung der Dehnbarkeit des Nerven durch temporäre Verkoppelung bei großen Defekten zum Zweck der Nervennaht. Bruns Beitr. klin. Chir. 105 (1917), 651—666.
Mumenthaler, M., Schliack, H.: Läsionen peripherer Nerven. Stuttgart: Thieme. 1965.
Naffziger, H. C.: Methods to secure end-to-end suture of peripheral nerves. Surg. Gynec. Obstet. 32 (1921), 193—204.
Nauck, E. Th.: Bemerkungen über den mechanisch-funktionellen Bau der Nerven. Anat. Anz., Erg. H. 72 (1931), 260—275.
Neri, V.: Die nervösen Folgeerscheinungen der einseitigen und doppelseitigen Ischiadicusdehnung. Experimentelle und klinische Studie. Z. orthop. Chir. 24 (1909), 87—104.
Nigst, H.: Die traumatische Neuritis des N. ulnaris. Eine Analyse von 73 operierten Fällen. Helv. chir. Acta 20 (1953), 37—51.
— Die Chirurgie der peripheren Nerven. Stuttgart: Thieme. 1955.
— Operative Behandlungsmöglichkeiten bei Erkrankungen und frischen Verletzungen peripherer Nerven. Langenbecks Arch. klin. Chir. 301 (1962), 855—864.
— Periphere Nerven. In: Lehrbuch der Chirurgie; ed. by Hellner, Nissen, and Vosschulte. Stuttgart: Thieme. 1964.
Nissl, F.: Über die Veränderungen der Ganglienzellen am Facialiskern des Kaninchens nach Ausreißung der Nerven. Allg. Z. Psychiat. 48 (1892), 197—198.
Olsson, Y.: Studies on vascular permeability in peripheral nerves. I. Distribution of circulating fluorescent serum albumin in normal, crushed and sectioned rat sciatic nerve. Acta Neuropath. (Berlin) 7 (1966), 1—15.
— The effect of the histamine liberator, compound 48/80 on mast cells in normal peripheral nerves. Acta path. mikrobiol. scand. 68 (1966), 575—584.
Ommaya, A. K.: Mechanical properties of tissues of the nervous system. J. Biomechanics 1 (1968), 127—138.
Pendl, O.: Die Weichteile des Bewegungsapparates. In: Handbuch der speziellen pathologischen Anatomie, ed. by Kaufmann, E., Staemmler, M., Bd. II/4. Berlin: W. de Gruyter & Co. 1963.
Penzholz: Diskussionsbemerkung. Symposium über Verletzungen peripherer Nerven. Kassel-Wilhelmshöhe, 3.—4. 2. 1972. Melsunger med. Mitt. 46, Heft 116 (1972), 161.
Petrov, M., Solarov, T.: Vortrag — 42. Tag. Bayer. Chirurgen-Vereinigung. Erlangen, 23.—24. 7. 1965.
— Nervenautoplastiken. Münch. med. Wschr. 108 (1966), 752—759.
Pia, H. W., Kunze, K., Miehlke, A., Mittelmeier, H., Penzholz, H., Puff, K. H., Rehn, J., Samii, M., Struppler, A.: Versorgung von Nervenverletzungen. Dtsch. Ärzteblatt 75 (1978), 565—577.
Piscol, K.: Histologischer Bau der peripheren Nerven, die histopathologischen Veränderungen bei Läsionen peripherer Nerven, Degeneration, Regeneration, Läsionstypen. In: Läsionen peripherer Nerven, ed. by Mumenthaler, M., H. Schliack. Stuttgart: Thieme. 1965.
Platt, H.: The surgery of peripheral nerve injuries of warfare. Brit. med. J. 1 (1921), 596—600.

Platt, H., Bristow, W. R.: The remote results of operations for injuries of the peripheral nerves. Brit. J. Surg. *11* (1923), 535—559.

Prevost, J. L.: Expériences rélatives à l'élongation des nerfs et aux névrites. Revue méd. Suisse romande *1* (1881), 469—489.

Quinquaud: Recherches sur l'élongation des nerfs. C. R. Soc. Biol. (Paris) *3* (1882), 119.

Rexed, B., Swennsson, A.: Über die Regeneration der Markscheide bei peripheren Nerven nach Kontinuitätstrennungen. Z. mikr.-anat. Forsch. *49* (1940), 359—387.

Ricker, G., Ellenbeck, J.: Beiträge zur Kenntnis der Veränderungen des Muskels nach der Durchschneidung seines Nerven. Virchows Arch. path. Anat. Physiol., klin. Med. *158* (1899), 199—253.

Röttgen, P.: Der heutige Stand der Chirurgie peripherer Nervenverletzungen. Zbl. Chir. *74* (1949), 406—407.

— Über traumatische und mechanische Nervenschäden. Landarzt *35* (1959), 186—191.

Samii, M.: Interfaszikuläre autologe Nerventransplantation. Dtsch. Ärzteblatt 1973, Heft *19*, 1257—1262.

— Modern aspects of peripheral and cranial nerve surgery. Advances and technical standards in neurosurgery. Vol. 2, pp. 33—85. Wien-New York: Springer. 1975.

— Kahl, R.-I.: Klinische Resultate der autologen Nerventransplantationen. Symposium über Verletzungen peripherer Nerven. Kassel-Wilhelmshöhe, 3.—4. 2. 1972. Melsunger Med. Mitt. *46*, Heft 116 (1972), 197—202.

— Scheinpflug, W.: Klinische, elektromyographische und quantitativ histologische Untersuchungen nach Nerventransplantationen. Acta Neurochir. (Wien) *30* (1974), 1—29.

— Schürmann, K., Wallenborn, R., Scheinpflug, W.: Tierexperimentelle Untersuchungen über autologe und homologe Nerventransplantationen. Symposium über Verletzungen peripherer Nerven. Kassel-Wilhelmshöhe, 3.—4. 2. 1972. Melsunger Med. Mitt. *46*, Heft 116 (1972), 333—339.

— Wallenborn, R.: Tierexperimentelle Untersuchungen über den Einfluß der Spannung auf den Regenerationserfolg nach Nervennaht. Acta Neurochir. (Wien) *27* (1972), 87—110.

— Willebrand, U.: Zur Indikation und Technik der interfaszikulären autologen Nerventransplantation. Vortr. Jahrestag. dtsch. Ges. Neurochir. 1970.

Sanders, F. K.: The repair of large gaps in the peripheral nerves. Brain *65* (1942), 281—337.

— The fate of nerve homografts in the rabbit. J. Anat. (Lond.) *83* (1949), 80.

— The preservation of nerve grafts. In: Preservation and Transplantation of normal Tissues. CIBA Found. Symp., London 1954.

— Young, J. Z.: The degeneration and re-innervation of grafted nerves. J. Anat. (Lond.) *76* (1942), 143—166.

— The role of the peripheral stump in the control of fibre diameter in regenerating nerves. J. Physiol. (Lond.) *103* (1944), 119—136.

Scarff, J. E.: The surgical treatment of injuries of the brain, spinal cord and peripheral nerves. Surg. Gynec. Obstet. *81* (1945), 405—424.

— Peripheral nerve injuries: Principles of treatment. Med. Clin. N. Amer. *42* (1958), 611—640.

Scheving, F.: De l'élongation des nerfs. Thèse de Paris 1881.

Schleich, G.: Versuche über die Reizbarkeit der Nerven im Dehnungszustand. Z. Biol. (München) *7* (1871), 379—394.

Schlote, W.: Morphologische und histochemische Untersuchungen an retrograden Axonveränderungen im Zentralnervensystem. Acta Neuropath. (Berlin) *1* (1961), 135—158.

Schneider, D.: Die Dehnbarkeit der markhaltigen Nervenfaser des Frosches in Abhängigkeit von Funktion und Struktur. Z. Naturforsch., B, *7* (1952), 38—48.

Scholz, W.: Regressive bzw. dystrophische Krankheitsprozesse, sogenannte Degenerationsprozesse und ihre Ausbreitung im Nervensystem. In: Handbuch der speziellen pathologischen Anatomie und Histologie, ed. by Henke-Lubarsch, Bd. XIII/1, 28 ff. Berlin-Göttingen-Heidelberg: Springer. 1957.

— Für die allgemeine Histopathologie degenerativer Prozesse bedeutsame morphologische, histochemische und strukturphysiologische Daten. In: Handbuch der speziellen pathologischen Anatomie und Histologie, ed. by Henke-Lubarsch, Bd. XIII/1, 43 ff. Berlin-Göttingen-Heidelberg: Springer. 1957.

— An nervöse Systeme gebundene (topistische) Kreislaufschäden. In: Handbuch der speziellen pathologischen Anatomie und Histologie, ed. by Henke-Lubarsch, Bd. XIII/1, 1326 ff. Berlin-Göttingen-Heidelberg: Springer. 1957.

— Die nicht zur Erweichung führenden unvollständigen Gewebsnekrosen (elektive Parenchymnekrosen). In: Handbuch der speziellen pathologischen Anatomie und Histologie, ed. by Henke-Lubarsch, Bd. XIII/1, 1284 ff. Berlin-Göttingen-Heidelberg: Springer. 1957.

Schröder, J. M., Seiffert, K. E.: Die Feinstruktur der neuromatösen Neurotisation von Nerventransplantaten. Virchows Arch. path. Anat., Abt. B, Zellpath. *5* (1970), 219—235.

Seddon, H. J.: Three types of nerve injury. Brain *66* (1943), 237—288.

— War injuries of peripheral nerves. Brit. J. Surg., War Surgery Suppl. No. 2, Wounds of the extremities, 1949, pp. 325—353.

— Peripheral nerve injuries. Med. Res. Council Spec. Rep. Series No. 282, London 1954.

— Nerve grafting. J. Bone Jt Surg. *45 B* (1963), 447—461.

Seiffert, K. E.: Diskussionsbemerkung. Symposium über Verletzungen peripherer Nerven. Kassel-Wilhelmshöhe, 3.—4. 2. 1972. Melsunger Med. Mitt. *46*, Heft 116 (1972), 160—161.

Seitelberger, F.: Zur Morphologie und Histochemie der degenerativen Axonveränderungen im Zentralnervensystem. III. Congr. Intern. Neuropath., Acta med. belg. 127—147, Brüssel 1957.

— Gross, H.: Über eine spätinfantile Form der Hallervorden-Spatzschen Krankheit. Dtsch. Z. Nervenheilk. *176* (1957), 104—125.

Slauck, A.: Beitrag zur Kenntnis der Muskelpathologie. Z. ges. Neurol. Psychiat. *71* (1921) 352—356.

— Histopathologische Untersuchungen bei neuraler Myopathie. Klin. Wschr. *2* (1928), 2245—2247.

— Pathologische Anatomie der Myopathien. In: Handbuch der Neurologie, ed. by Bumke and Foerster, Bd. XVI, 412 ff. Berlin: Springer. 1936.

Smith, J. W.: Microsurgery of peripheral nerves. Plast. reconstr. Surg. *33* (1964), 317—329.

— Factors influencing nerve repair. Arch. Surg. *93* (1966), 335—341.

Spatz, H.: Über die Vorgänge nach experimenteller Rückenmarksdurchtrennung mit besonderer Berücksichtigung der Unterschiede der Reaktionsweise des reifen und unreifen Gehirns nebst Beziehungen zur menschlichen Pathologie (Porencephalie und Syringomyelie). Nissl-Alzheim. histol. Arb. Großhirnrinde, Bd. 6/Erg. 49 (1921), 364—355.

Spurling, R. G.: The use of tantalum wire and foil in the repair of peripheral nerves. Surg. Clin. N. Amer. *23* (1943), 1491—1504.
— Peripheral nerve injuries in European theatre of operations. Management with special reference to early nerve surgery. J. Amer. med. Ass. *129* (1945), 1011—1014.
Stintzing, R.: Über Nervendehnung; eine experimentelle und klinische Studie. Leipzig: Vogel. 1883.
Stoffel, A.: Über Nervenmechanik und ihre Bedeutung für die Behandlung der Nervenverletzungen. Münch. med. Wschr. *62* (1915), 889—892.
Stookey, B.: Surgical and mechanical treatment of peripheral nerves. Philadelphia: Saunders Co. 1922.
Sunderland, S.: The effect of rupture of the perineurium on the contained nervefibres. Brain *69* (1946), 149—152.
— The connective tissues of peripheral nerves. Brain *88* (1965), 841—854.
— Nerves and nerve injuries. Edinburgh-London: Churchill Livingstone. 1972.
— Denervation atrophy of the distal stump of a severed nerve. J. comp. Neurol. *93* (1950), 401—409.
— Bradley, K. C.: Endoneurial tube shrinkage in the distal segment of a severed nerve. J. comp. Neurol. *93* (1950), 411—420.
— The perineurium of peripheral nerves. Anat. Rec. *113* (1952), 125—141.
— Stress-strain phenomena in human peripheral nerve trunks. Brain *84* (1961), 102—119.
— Stress-strain phenomena in human spinal nerve roots. Brain *84* (1961), 120—124.
— Stress-strain phenomena in denervated peripheral nerve trunks. Brain *84* (1961), 125—127.
Swan, J.: Discussion on injuries to the peripheral nerves. Proc. roy. Soc. Med. *34* (1941), 521—529.
Symington, J.: The physics of nerve stretching. Brit. med. J. *1* (1882), 770—771.
Takimoto, G.: Über die Nervendehnung. Experimentelle und klinische Untersuchung. Mitt. med. Fak. K. jap. Univ. *16* (1916), 73—136.
Tarnomsky: Cited by Takimoto, G., 1916.
Terzis, J., Faibisoff, B., Williams, H. B.: The nerve gap: Suture under tension vs. graft. Plast. reconstr. Surg. *56* (1975), 166—170.
Thomas, P. K., Jones, D. G.: The cellular response to nerve injury. II. Regeneration of the perineurium after nerve section. J. Anat. (Lond.) *101* (1967), 45—55.
Thomson, J. L., Ritchie, W. P., French, L. A., Wrork, D. W.: Plan for the care of peripheral nerve injuries overseas. Arch. Surg. (Chic.) *52* (1946), 557—570.
Thulin, C. A., Carlsson, C. A. (1969): Cited by Erbslöh, F., Hager, H.: Sekundäre Muskelveränderungen bei peripheren Nervenläsionen. Symposium über Verletzungen peripherer Nerven. Kassel-Wilhelmshöhe, 3.—4. 2. 1972. Melsunger Med. Mitt. *46*, Heft 116 (1972), 53—83.
Tillaux, P.: Des affections chirurgicales des nerfs. Thesis. P. Asselin, Paris 1866.
Trombetta, F.: Sullo stiramento dei nervi; studi patologici e clinici. Messina: Frat. d'Angelo. 1880.
Valentin, G.: Versuch einer physiologischen Pathologie der Nerven, Part 2. Leipzig-Heidelberg: Winter. 1864.
— Berliner Verein für innere Medicin. Discussion. Dtsch. med. Wschr. *7* (1881), 46—47,
Verneuil: Dehnung bei Tetanus. Erfolg. Brit. med. J. *18*, Vol. II (1876), 173.
Vogt, P.: Die Nerven-Dehnung als Operation in der chirurgischen Praxis; eine experimentelle und klinische Studie. Leipzig: Vogel. 1877.

Wagner, H.: Operative Beinverlängerung. Chirurg *42* (1971), 260—266.

Wechsler, W., Hager, H.: Elektronenmikroskopische Befunde am atrophischen quergestreiften Skelettmuskel der Ratte nach Nervdurchtrennung. Naturwissensch. 47 (1960), 185—186.

— Elektronenmikroskopische Befunde an der quergestreiften Skelettmuskulatur bei spinaler Muskelatrophie. Naturwissensch. *47* (1960), 604—605.

— Elektronenmikroskopische Befunde bei Muskelatrophie nach Nervendurchtrennung bei der weißen Ratte. Beitr. path. Anat. *125* (1961), 31—53.

— Elektronenmikroskopische Befunde zur Feinstruktur von Axonveränderungen regenerierender Nervenfasern im Nervus ischiadicus der weißen Ratte. Acta Neuropath. (Berlin) *1* (1962), 489—506.

— Elektronenmikroskopische Untersuchung der sekundären Wallerschen Degeneration des peripheren Säugetiernerven. Beitr. path. Anat. *126* (1962), 352—380.

Weddell, G.: Axonal regeneration in cutaneous nerve plexuses. J. Anat. (Lond.) *77* (1942), 49—62.

Weiss, P.: Sutureless reunion of severed nerves with elastic cuffs of tantalum. J. Neurosurg. *1* (1944), 219—225.

— The technology of nerve regeneration: A review. Sutureless tubulation and related methods of nerve repair. J. Neurosurg. *1* (1944), 400—450.

— Damming of axoplasm in constricted nerves: A sign of perpetual growth in nerve fibres. Anat. Rec. *88* (1944), 464—479.

— Experiments on cell and axon orientation in vitro: The role of colloidal exudates in tissue organization. J. exp. Zool. *100* (1945), 353—386.

Whitcomb, B. B.: Separation at the suture site as a cause of failure in regeneration of peripheral nerves. J. Neurosurg. *3* (1946), 399—406.

Witkowski, L.: Zur Nervendehnung. Arch. Psychiat. Nervenkr. *11* (1881), 532—537.

Wohlfart, G.: Degenerative and regenerative axonal changes in the ventral horns, brain stem and cerebral cortex in amyotrophic lateral sclerosis. Lunds Universitets Arsskrift. N. F. Avd. 2, *56*, Nr. 2, 3—13, Lund 1959.

Woodhall, B.: The zone of interior. Chapter 10 in Medical Department, United States Army, Surgery in World War II, Neurosurgery, Vol. 2, Part II, Peripheral nerve injuries, ed. by Spurling, R. G., Woodhall, B. Washington, D.C.: US Government Printing Office. 1959.

Young, J. Z.: The functional repair of nervous tissue. Physiol. Rev. *22* (1942), 318—374.